DOES IT HURT?

DOES IT HURT?

A Dialog to Help You Understand and Trust Acupuncture

A. Burton Moomaw, LAc. DiplAc.

DOES IT HURT PUBLISHING, LLC • BOONE, NC

Printed in the United States of America

DOES IT HURT PUBLISHING, LLC

Moomaw, A. Burton
Does it hurt?: a dialog to help you understand and trust acupuncture / A. Burton
Moomaw

ISBN 978-0-578-55120-3   Non-fiction
1. Acupressure & Acupuncture 2. Alternative Therapies 3. Pain Management

Cover Design by Courtney Tiberio
Interior Layout by Susan Yost
Photography by Todd Bush Photography

To view full-color versions of the images in this book, visit:
www.BooneAcupuncture.com/color-images.

Dedicated to Bud Harris
for his love, wisdom, and guidance.

Disclaimer

This book is intended for informational and educational purposes only. It should not be interpreted as medical advice to readers attempting to diagnose and treat their own illnesses. It is the reader's responsibility to seek out an expert diagnosis and treatment for any health concern by consulting trained, medical professionals. The author makes no explicit or implicit guarantees that acupuncture will help any given medical condition. *Does It Hurt?* is offered to the uninitiated as an introduction to an alternative method of medical treatment besides the conventional system of modern medicine most familiar to us in the U.S.

Table of Contents

Note: To view full-color versions of the images in this book, visit: www.BooneAcupuncture.com/color-images.

I desire that the citizens of my kingdom be prevented from using toxic remedies, using instead only the fine needles.

— Huangdi

The Yellow Emperor, 2800 bce

INTRODUCTION

ACUPUNCTURE is a medical healing art which uses solid, hair-thin needles inserted into the skin and muscles to aid the body in correcting health problems.

There is no concept in modern medical science that can explain how acupuncture works. It does not stimulate the nervous system to cause a healing effect. It does not release endorphins to eliminate pain. Acupuncture needles activate the flow of energy throughout the body in our Energetic System. How this happens can only be understood and assessed from the viewpoint of the qualitative science from which it evolved.

Daoist philosophy developed the organizational models that describe energy and acupuncture. Acupuncturists assess the whole person using Yin/Yang, Five Phases, Energetic Channels, and Pulse and Tongue Diagnosis. These models help them synthesize all physical and emotional symptoms manifesting in the body into a single diagnostic picture.

Based on this diagnosis, the relevant acupuncture points on the appropriate channels are treated with needles to stimulate the body's energy which directs the function of the entire system. The stimulation of this energy activates the body's own ability to return to a state of health and displace or eradicate disease. Your Energetic System reaches every part of your being—body, mind, and spirit. Therefore, acupuncture can be used to treat an extremely wide range of health issues from pain to digestion to depression.

This book is a synthesis of the organizational models and concepts of Chinese medicine presented in simple terms I use with each of my patients. It is written for those with a newfound curiosity about the topic. As with any unfamiliar concept, even the simplest description can seem complex and strange at first. My goal is to remove some of the mystery surrounding acupuncture and provide you with a broader understanding of this alternative way to improve your health.

The impetus to write this book came from my desire to share the amazing changes I see in my patients on a daily basis. I've witnessed a veteran's leg pain subside by 70% during the first treatment, a man's 37-year-old headache resolve and remain gone for two years after a course of treatments, and a young cancer patient's appetite return after needling only one acupuncture point. I am grateful to have assisted these powerful experiences of self-healing, and firmly believe that acupuncture should be the first-line treatment for many health issues.

During my first decade as an acupuncturist, I noticed certain questions were repeatedly posed by new patients or others curious about the topic. I have taken this cue and organized the following Frequently Asked Questions into chapters sequenced as they are typically asked. I believe this serves as an approachable introduction for the uninitiated, and a natural evolution of the material.

Does It Hurt?: A Dialog to Help You Understand and Trust Acupuncture is intended for both healthcare consumers and providers, since members from both of these groups have expressed a great deal of interest in the topic to me. I trust that the concepts described herein will demystify this ancient model of medicine, and serve as a useful resource.

The doctor of the future will give no medicine, but will interest his patient in the care of the human body, in diet, and in the cause and prevention of disease.

— THOMAS EDISON (1847-1931)

CHAPTER I

Does It Hurt?

The first question I am asked about acupuncture is, "Does it hurt?"

I understand this concern, especially since acupuncture is most widely recognized as a treatment for pain. Honestly, from my own experience being treated and my experience giving over 15,000 treatments in the past 11 years, the answer is a resounding YES. You should, and do, feel the needles. But do read on; it is not nearly as scary as it may sound.

Acupuncture can be perceived as painful but, depending on your level of sensitivity, the sensation can vary. Some patients feel a light prick. Others may feel nothing at all. External factors such as time of day, season, or weather, can influence the level of sensation. Why does it hurt at all, and why the variation? Chinese medical theory offers some interesting explanations.

Acupuncture affects the body's function and health through energy. Energy is that non-physical part of us that directs our body functions. There are three types of energy: Yuan Chi, Ying Chi, and Wei Chi.

We feel the outside world with our Wei Chi, or defensive energy. It logically follows that Wei Chi is highly concentrated in the dermal layer of our skin as protection from outside pathogens. The presence of Wei Chi in our skin also allows us to feel a range of sensations from the excruciating bite of a dog, to the tickle from a blade of grass brushing against our skin, to the subtlest sensation of a breeze caressing our face. Naturally, we would feel the prick of an acupuncture needle.

Why do we feel pain when an outside force is strong enough to hurt us? Pain is a necessary part of our immune reaction. As defensive energy implies, Wei Chi signals the body to retreat from further attack by generating a pain sensation causing us to retract from the offense. Pain is necessary for survival.

How intense is the pain we feel from an acupuncture needle? Most describe what they feel as similar to a mosquito bite in intensity and duration. Others describe it as a pinch. Rarely, maybe one in 10,000 treatments, has a patient been unable to tolerate their sensation of pain from my needles.

I have introduced many people with trypanophobia, or a fear of needles, to their first experience with an acupuncture needle. Not once did someone say "Ouch, that hurt!" Most commonly they say, "Oh, it's in already? That's it?" A patient once said, "They really shouldn't be called needles. They are nothing like a hypodermic needle. They should be called filaments or wire filaments."

Acupuncture needles are made of stainless steel surgical wire tapered to a point. Like a syringe, they must be sterile before use and, by law, discarded after one insertion. The acupuncture needle design allows it to burrow between tissue fibers instead of severing them. They are inserted using a plastic tube that is slightly shorter than the needle. (See Figs. 1 and 2.) This facilitates entry through the skin, bypassing pain receptors, and causing little to no pain or bleeding.

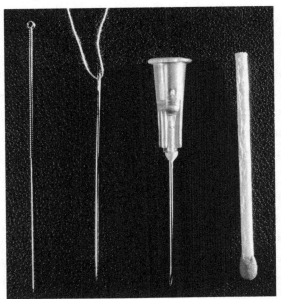

Fig. 1 Needle size comparison

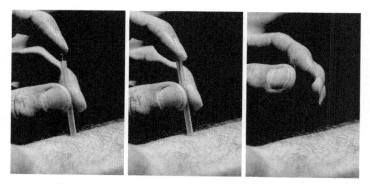

Fig. 2 Inserting the acupuncture needle with tube

In contrast, a hypodermic needle is a hollow tube with a razor-sharp, beveled tip which allows it to penetrate skin or the dense mantle of blood vessels. It has to be large enough and remain inserted long enough to transport fluids to and from the body. Most patients' needle fears come from past traumatic experiences of painful shots using hypodermic needles received in the doctor's office.

Inserting an acupuncture needle produces a sensation called Deqi—the arrival of the energy—which is the needle causing energy to move in its channel. The effect of the treatment is enhanced when Deqi occurs, so often your acupuncturist will move the needle in different ways to elicit its presence. The nature of the sensation can feel like a mild tingling at the needle site or radiating out a limb, a sensation felt somewhere else in the body, or an electrical feeling like when you hit your funny bone.

Deqi occurs sometime after the initial needle insertion. It is a fleeting sensation and does not persist. Many patients think that Deqi is a nerve being stimulated by the needle. If this were true, the sensation would persist until the needle was removed. If you ever feel persistent pain during an acupuncture treatment, ask your acupuncturist to adjust or remove the needle. You don't have to lie there and take it.

During my years of practice I have noticed a tremendous variation in the sensations that my patients experience—from needle to needle, within the same treatment, and from day to day. I attribute these variations to:

1. Each person's unique makeup and their current distribution of energy
2. Where on their body an acupuncture point is located
3. Seasonal and weather influence

1. Individual makeup

An underlying principle of Chinese medicine is individualization of each treatment. We are each unique in our state of being from minute to minute throughout the day. Each treatment should be approached by the acupuncturist as if it were a blank slate. This means that while one patient might never receive the same treatment twice, another patient might receive the same treatment every month for a year. Individual makeup also means that the same illness in two patients can manifest differently and therefore must be treated differently.

Our individuality means that each person has a unique distribution of energy throughout his/her body at any given moment. Returning to our topic of the sensation of pain, we feel the world with our Wei Chi. Wei Chi is hot and volatile, rushing instantly to the location it is called to for defense or repair. At various times of day it is concentrated in different parts of our body—mostly on the exterior during midday when the sun is strongest, and mostly in the interior during midnight to repair any damage from the day's metabolism.

Other factors that affect the status and location of our Wei Chi include our general state of health, our hydration level, and our current emotional state. When we are sick or dehydrated, our Wei Chi is taxed, preoccupied, and less able to defend us. This is why we are taught to drink plenty of fluids and to rest or relax when we are sick. When we are angry or stressed, our Wei Chi sits at the surface defending us from the emotional assault we are experiencing. We are more pain-sensitive when our Wei Chi is overactive at the surface or weakened by illness.

2. Location of the acupuncture point on your body
Different parts of our body experience different levels of sensation. In general, our torso feels less than our head

and limbs. We perceive the world through our five senses. We touch with our extremities, so there is more Wei Chi in our limbs than in our trunk. Similarly, Wei Chi activates our senses of sight, hearing, smell, and taste so we are alert to our surroundings. Physiologically this is comparable to the greater concentration of pain receptors located in our hands, feet, and face than in other parts of our body.

As a result, my patients often report more pain sensation from acupuncture needles placed in their hands, feet, and face. However, this does not always hold true for everyone. I have had patients who are more sensitive on their torso than their hands and feet, and others who simply experience more pain in parts of their bodies where they feel particularly vulnerable. Due to our individuality, each person can expect to experience his or her own unique perception of and sensation from acupuncture.

3. Seasonal and weather factors

Chinese medicine recognizes that humans are part of the natural world. Just as the earth has climates that vary from season to season, we too have an internal climate that changes with these cycles. External seasonal change requires our energy to respond, especially our Wei Chi.

In summer, we are more active. Heat generates a lot of activity in nature. Warmth is less difficult for most of us to adapt to since our internal climate is inherently warm. In summer our Wei Chi is less needed at the surface, but is paradoxically more available. Because of this, I have noticed that patients tend to feel a little more pain sensation from needles in the summer.

Winter's cold temperatures are a struggle for our warm bodies. Our Wei Chi is required at the surface to protect us from the cold, but it is less available because our bodies conserve heat by contracting our energy inward. With less Wei Chi at the surface, external cold can penetrate the surface channels in what is called a wind/cold invasion, otherwise known as the common cold. This is why cold and flu season occurs during fall, winter, and spring when outside temperatures drop to their lowest points. Less Wei Chi means less pain sensation from needles in winter.

Weather affects the level of needle sensation. There are days when virtually everyone I treat flinches when the needles go in. I'm quite certain that my needle technique does not change on those days. Needle sensitivity seems to occur most frequently on days of low barometric pressure associated with weather fronts. Once, we had two days of rain as a cold front passed through. On the second day, several patients, who had not previously experienced any pain from needle insertion, reacted several times.

IN SUMMARY:

- We are meant to feel sensations like pain as part of our defense system.
- Pain is an alarm to get us to pay attention.
- Most patients report that they feel very little sensation of pain from acupuncture needles.
- There are differences between hypodermic and acupuncture needles that contribute to the latter being less painful.
- Acupuncture needles create secondary sensation after insertion, called Deqi—the arrival of the energy. The sensation does not persist during treatment.
- There are many factors that affect the sensation you feel when an acupuncture needle penetrates your skin.

CHAPTER 2

Where Will You Put the Needles?

Often during their first visit to the acupuncturist, patients are concerned not only with whether the needles will hurt, but also how many needles will be used, and where they will be inserted. Some may envision their entire body covered in needles, or have fears about needling sensitive areas where they may feel vulnerable. These are all natural concerns. In reality, very few needles are required in a given treatment, and may be localized to a specific area of the body. There are also multiple needleless treatment options if someone is particularly sensitive to or afraid of a needle application to a particular area.

Each acupuncture treatment is uniquely tailored to the specific patient in the present moment. Treatments are determined not only by symptoms, but also by underlying causes of physical or emotional health. Both of these considerations influence which channels will be targeted during the treatment, and which points on those channels will receive a needle.

Acupuncture channels represent the circulatory system of our Energy. These channels deliver blueprint information, nourishment and protection to every cell in our body. Channels start in our head or torso and end at the tips of our fingers and toes. They have access to our entire internal landscape, including all of our vital organs. (See Fig. 3.)

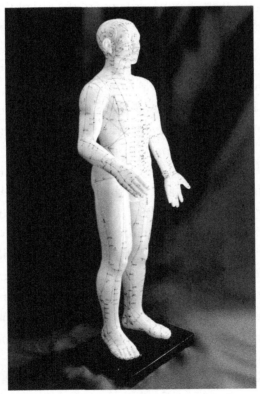

Fig. 3 Mannequin showing channels head to toe

It may be surprising to learn that needles are not necessarily inserted directly at the points where symptoms or pain occur. This is because channels traverse the body, like a roadmap, from the limbs all the way into the organs. Therefore, a needle placed in the liver channel in the foot can influence the function of the liver. That same needle would also be effective in a treatment for certain headaches because the liver channel also goes to the top of the head.

Assessing the underlying causes of a health problem can also influence where needles are placed. Continuing the previous example, the acupuncture point on the liver channel in the foot could be used for a patient whose headache is caused by malfunction with their liver energy or in the liver organ. But not all headaches are caused by problems with the liver energy. A patient with a headache caused by wind/cold might be needled on their fourth toe and on their head where the pain actually exists. This targets the gallbladder channel in order to release trapped pathogenic energy.

There is no way to generalize where needles will be placed for a given condition. This decision must be made at the moment of treatment guided by the patient's emotional state, physical signs and symptoms, and other diagnostic criteria from the organizational models of Chinese medicine.

Since the energy channels traverse every inch of our body, there is some flexibility in choosing where the needles will go. If a patient is anxious about having a needle placed in the liver channel in their foot, I can choose an alternative point on the liver channel in their abdomen to help alleviate their headache.

Healing is a collaborative process between a patient and his/her healthcare provider. Most patients are infinitely more familiar with the depths of their physical and emotional struggles than I am. Therefore, involving them in the execution of their own care regimen is essential for improvement. Communication is key to guiding the course I will take with the treatment, as I want to respect any apprehensions my patient may feel. Together we will find the most comfortable needle combination for each treatment.

CASE STUDY

A new patient, a 10-year-old boy, came in for treatment one day. He was excited about the experience and naturally wondered if it would hurt, how many needles I would use, and where I would put them. After taking his medical history and considering his current symptoms, I formed a diagnosis and treatment plan.

I told him I had chosen four points to needle: two on his torso, one on his leg, and one on his foot. I explained that the needles inserted into the trunk of his body would likely hurt less than the ones on his leg and foot, and suggested that we start with the point above his belly button. This point I considered most important because of its effect on several energy channels.

He was pleasantly surprised by how little discomfort he felt from this needle and agreed to continue with the second one near his shoulder. Again, he felt very little discomfort, but noticed the secondary sensation of Deqi (the arrival of energy) at the needle. He agreed to a third needle, inserted just below his knee. From this one, he felt a slightly more painful sensation, and at that point decided he did not want to have the fourth needle placed in his foot. Instead, I activated the point with acupressure and warmed it with a heat source called Moxa.

Allowing the boy to have input and the final word in his treatment not only contributed to his overall comfort level with the process, but also made him aware that options besides needles exist which can achieve the desired effect. By his third treatment he had grown accustomed to the needle sensation, and asked for the needle in his foot.

Alternatives to Needling

The following therapeutic methods may be used in place of or in addition to needles in the same treatment session.

Moxa is an herb called mugwort rolled up in paper like a cigar, or placed as balls on top of a needle. It is burned and used to slowly warm acupuncture points from a distance of about two inches. The warmth adds yang energy to your channels to enhance internal function. Moxa is used in cases of cold conditions, but never for heat or inflammation. (See Fig. 4.)

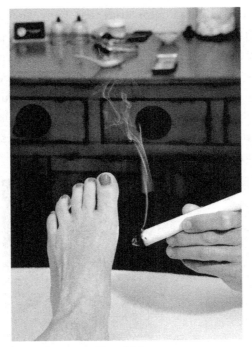

Fig. 4 Moxa

Gua Sha is a technique that uses a Chinese soup spoon or other utensil to scrape the skin and release stagnation at the surface. "Gua" means scraping. "Sha" is the deep-red to purple blotching that appears on the skin from scraping, and is the physical manifestation of the release of blockage in painful areas. Gua Sha allows energy and blood to recirculate, reducing pain. (See Fig. 5.)

Cupping was brought to public attention during the 2016 Summer Olympic Games when the champion swimmer Michael Phelps appeared with purple circles across his back. In cupping, suction cups that pull outward on the channels are placed on areas of soreness. Just like Gua Sha, the decompression of the channel releases stagnant energy and restores circulation. The cup marks are not bruising. They are Sha—stagnation dissipating at the surface. Both cup marks and Sha disappear within hours to a few days. (See Fig. 6.)

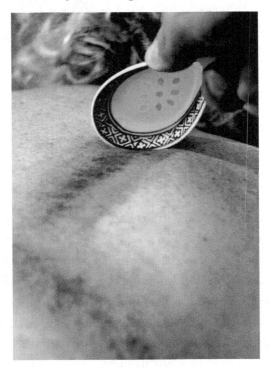

Fig. 5 Gua Sha

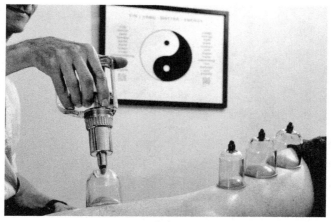

Fig. 6 Cupping

Acupressure (applying pressure to acupuncture points) with a finger has the same effect as inserting needles. It activates the point, thereby influencing the energy in the channel.

Electrical Stimulation uses a microcurrent of electricity to stimulate the point. The current may be induced using a small hand-held electrical device placed on a point and triggered for a few seconds (See Fig. 7.), or a larger device, attached by leads to acupuncture needles, may be used to deliver a current for a longer period of time. (See Fig. 8.) This method is sometimes used in cases of severe pain or for pain control during surgery.

Finally, for those with a paralyzing fear of the idea of a needle placed in your skin and remaining there, needles are not absolutely necessary for an effective acupuncture treatment.

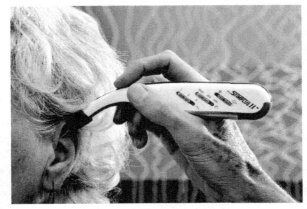

Fig. 7 Hand-held electrical device

I have performed treatments on both children and adults using one or a combination of the techniques listed above to stimulate acupuncture points. I have seen only minor differences in the effectiveness of these treatments. I encourage you to work with your acupuncturist to find the type of point stimulation right for you. Over time, the treatments will allay any heightened fear about your body and the potential for pain from needles.

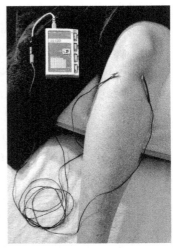

Fig. 8 Electrical stimulation

IN SUMMARY:

- The number of needles and where they are placed may vary with each treatment.
- There is flexibility in points chosen for treatment because the channels traverse the entire body.
- Vulnerable parts of your body do not absolutely have to receive a needle.
- Communication with your acupuncturist about needle location and number will help minimize your concern.
- There are alternatives to needles that are equally effective.
- Gua Sha, Cupping and Moxa are frequently incorporated into acupuncture treatments.

CHAPTER 3

Does It Work?

There is a fair amount of skepticism in Western cultures regarding the legitimacy and effectiveness of traditional Chinese medicine. In the United States especially, the majority's only recourse for addressing health problems has historically been some version of the contemporary practice evolved from 18th century European medical science. From this indoctrination, we generally follow two basic treatments for all illnesses:

1. PHARMACOLOGY – applying, ingesting or injecting a chemical drug to correct an imbalance.
2. SURGERY – cutting out the offending organ or tissue.

It can be a difficult leap for some to accept that simple micro-needles with no chemical substance in or on them, inserted into invisible channels in the body, can change our health too. It seems like magic, which doesn't sit well with the rational, material, quantitative understanding of our bodies we are more familiar with.

Chinese Medicine vs. Modern Medicine

Modern medicine is generally attributed to Hippocrates of ancient Greece (c. 460 BCE). The hallmark of his theory of medicine was that disease is caused naturally, meaning physically, by factors in the surrounding environment. Until Hippocrates, most cultures believed that the cause of disease was supernatural, coming from superstition or gods.

It was not until the late 18th and 19th centuries that Hippocrates' ideas began to flourish in Western culture. Significant discoveries and advancements were made that remain cornerstones of modern medicine today: vaccination, antibiotics, antiseptics, genetics, and more. Louis Pasteur (1822-1895), one of the founders of microbiology, and his colleagues were the first to research bacteria, its origin in the environment around us, and its potential to make us sick. This is the germ theory of disease from which the disease-management approach of modern medicine developed.

Claude Bernard (1813-1878) was the first scientist to describe the *milieu interieur*, the internal functional state of autoregulation in biological beings.[1] This is what modern medicine calls homeostasis.

Homeostasis is the concept that physiologically our bodies adjust their internal function automatically.

---

1 Daniel Murrell, MD, rev., "What is Modern Medicine?", *Medical News Today* (Oct. 31, 2018): www.medicalnewstoday.com.

These continual adjustments allow us to function while reacting to constant bombardment from the outside environment. This includes our ongoing response to physical toxins and germs.

The two organizational models of modern medicine, 1) Anatomy and Physiology and 2) Pathophysiology, divide the body into different systems, then delineate the diseases that affect each system. Specialists study specific branches of medicine relating to these systems: dermatology, neurology, dentistry, otorhinolaryngology, cardiology, gastroenterology, orthopedics, ophthalmology, hematology, hepatology, podiatry, psychiatry, obstetrics and gynecology, urology, immunology, oncology, etc. More general knowledge is held by family practice physicians and internists. The sheer volume of analytical information about function and treatment is so vast that few doctors can retain the details of all of these specialties.

Modern medicine is a system of disease diagnosis and management. Its study first involves learning human anatomy and physiology, the study of our physical body and its function in a healthy state. Next comes pathophysiology, the study of disease. Medical school curriculum requires intense memorization of the signs and symptoms of disease. Aligning the signs and symptoms with the results of different medical tests leads to a diagnosis of a named disease.

There is great emphasis in this diagnostic process

on the use of material measurement. Blood analysis and internal imaging are two examples. Treatment options in modern medicine include application, ingestion or injection of pharmaceuticals, surgery on the diseased body part, and physical therapy.

In modern medicine there is a clear focus on physical disease. The quantification of human anatomy and physiology and pathophysiology has created a systematized, rational, analytical approach to our health.

To a large degree, modern medicine separates emotional/mental health from physical health. Up to this point in the progression of material science, there is no way to establish a link between the two. Emotional/mental health usually is not assessed as part of physical disease. This is rooted in modern science's focus on measurable quantities. Psychiatry focuses on a chemical explanation of emotions. Neurology tries to quantify areas of the brain related to emotions, but since emotional/mental health cannot be quantified, it does not fit neatly into any numerical science model. It has been passed on to the qualitative field of psychology.

The strength of modern medicine lies in its treatment of acute illness and traumatic injury. There is no better option for addressing critical and life-threatening health issues. I am grateful that I could go to a hospital for emergency care when I broke my leg in high school, and when my heart stopped briefly later in life.

Chinese Medicine

Acupuncture is based on medical theory developed within the ancient Chinese philosophy of Daoism (c. 400 BCE). There is evidence that acupuncture has been in continuous use, treating one fifth of the world's population, for at least 2,000 years. Acupuncture received significant exposure in the United States in 1972 after a *New York Times* article was written on the subject by a journalist who accompanied President Richard Nixon on his historic trip to China. Over the last several decades, the practice has grown in popularity. Today there are acupuncture licensing boards in 48 states. Thousands of private practices can be found throughout the country. Acupuncturists work in hospitals and Department of Veterans Affairs facilities, and treatments are even covered by insurance in some states.

Daoist philosophy incorporated a scientific inquiry of nature best called Daoist physics. It involves intensive study of natural phenomena on the macro-scale, visible to the human eye, over hundreds of years. The great distinction of Daoism is its use of qualitative assessment and description. This means examining the essential nature of a subject and describing it in non-material ways.

Take, for example, a rainbow trout. Qualitatively it is an animal that lives immersed in water, moves elegantly with side-to-side articulation of its body, has fan-like appendages on its sides, back, and tail, and is colored greenish-brown with a stripe on its side that resembles a rainbow. Quantitatively, a rainbow trout is an aquatic, cold-blooded vertebrate of the genus Salmanoid. Its average weight is one to five pounds. It has five fins, and it breathes using two sets of gills to extract oxygen from the water. Each approach describes the trout in unique ways.

In relation to human health, qualitative science logically assumes that human beings are part of nature and, therefore, the same principles apply, only on a smaller scale. This is the concept of microcosm and macrocosm. The human being is a small but complete system (microcosm) within and identical to the grand system (macrocosm) of nature.

Do these qualitative concepts of human health overlap with modern medical quantitative ideas? Absolutely. Following acupuncture treatments, I have seen my patients' blood work improve, X-ray images of a non-healing fracture change dramatically, and eye pressure from glaucoma decrease substantially. Acupuncture simply affects human health by acting on an aspect undetectable by modern science—our Energetic System.

For seven years during and after acupuncture school, I had the privilege of studying with Dr. Tran Viet Tzung, a French medical doctor. He gave up his practice as a surgeon in Paris after he was introduced to acupuncture by his mentor Dr. Nguyen Van Nghi. Together they translated several ancient Chinese medical texts.

Through their collective lens of modern medical training, they recognized that the 2,000-year-old qualitative descriptions in the ancient medical texts were the same as the quantitative concepts of modern medicine. Dr. Tran felt that the astute material observations of modern science gave him conviction about the succinct qualitative descriptions of ancient Chinese medical theory.

My favorite way to describe the intersection of Chinese and modern medicine comes from Dr. Tran. He said, "If you look out the window and see a leaf moving on a tree, what is causing it to move?" Think about this for a minute. Outside of a direct external force acting on the leaf, such as a squirrel or earth tremor physically shaking the branch or the tree, the leaf is most likely moved by the wind.

Can you take a bottle, capture the wind, and hand it to me so that I can open the bottle and experience the breeze? No. We know that wind exists from our experience of it. We can measure its speed and direction, but we can't quantify it. No weather forecast ever predicted three million cubic feet of wind to blow through your town. Wind is a qualitative phenomenon that is very real, but not easily measured or described quantitatively.

Tran continues, "The moving leaf, this is modern medicine. The wind, this is Chinese medicine." Like the wind moving the leaf, we too have an invisible system moving our physical and emotional selves. Our "wind" is Chi, or energy.

I realize that the concept of centuries-old qualitative assessment and non-material treatment for modern day health issues sounds strange, especially in this era of rapid technological advancement. However, if you really examine how you assess the world minute-by-minute, you will see that it is almost all qualitative. You do not describe your day by saying, "I had three bushels of happiness today." You say, "I felt really happy today." This is a qualitative assessment. It is the reduction of our biology into quantifiable parts that has led us to expect the measurement of our health to be by the numbers only.

What led us to seek a rational explanation of our health in the first place? It is the nature of the human mind to seek out and define causes and effects in the world as a means of safety, prediction and organization. We get satisfaction from solutions to problems that fit in nice, neat, little boxes. Qualitative phenomena, like unusual weather or extreme behavior, scare us because they cannot be readily quantified, predicted or explained away.

So how do we know if acupuncture works when it is based on immeasurable theory? From my practice treating patients for more than a decade, I know it works. I have empirical data, anecdotal evidence, and years of observing medical data before and after treatments that have convinced me. Absence of numerical data does not negate my or my patients' experience. We would be foolish not to take advantage of the potential of energetic medicine while we wait for "hard science" to satisfy our intellectual needs. I am fortunate and grateful to have witnessed the effectiveness of this medicinal art that has helped patients ranging in age from three months to 94 years.

Acupuncture has been so widely accepted as an alternative treatment in human medicine that it has been applied in veterinary medicine as well. As we know, animals cannot tell you what they feel, so they are not subject to the placebo effect—a favored explanation by acupuncture's detractors for its unexplainable effect in humans. When animals get better from acupuncture treatments, it is not as easily explained away as being "all in their head."

If acupuncture didn't work, it wouldn't be in such high demand by our war veterans who suffer some of the worst cases of pain and trauma known. The U.S. Department of Veterans Affairs now employs acupuncturists and, due to high demand, is contracting with outside service providers to meet the need. Veterans' testaments that acupuncture works when the medications don't is not to be taken lightly.

CASE STUDY

Very early in my practice I began working with a 32-year-old woman. She came to me with pain and stiffness in her neck, the result of whiplash from an automobile accident. She had heard of acupuncture as an alternative treatment for pain. As I collected her medical history, she asked if I thought acupuncture could also help with gastroparesis. This condition is a severe malfunction of the stomach with partial paralysis that causes great difficulty with digestion. I told her there was great potential it would help, but explained that acupuncture is not magic. However, there are clear treatment principles that, when applied, could help coax her stomach to function properly. I told her healing is a process. It can take time and regular treatments to make a difference. She committed to come in twice a week for a month, then weekly after that as needed.

Part of this patient's personal history included a highly competitive childhood, schooling, and career. Her stomach problem started when she entered the stressful environment of graduate school. She sought help from modern medicine for four years, consulting some of the best gastroenterology specialists on the East Coast. She was ultimately presented with the option of having a gastric pacemaker implanted to stimulate her stomach electrically when one of the specialists suggested she try acupuncture first.

I distinctly remember my amazement when, during the first treatment, her stomach made a rumbling, hunger sound. After nine acupuncture treatments, she returned to her gastroenterologist for tests. The results showed that her stomach function had returned to 100%.

This patient continued with randomly-spaced rounds of treatment for eight more years. Acupuncture has helped her neck pain, pituitary dysfunction, fertility, and chronic psoriasis. She also credits acupuncture with a newfound ability to examine her life and make difficult but meaningful lifestyle changes which have greatly reduced her stress level and improved her general physical health.

Her Chinese medical diagnosis was cold in her stomach due to deficient kidney fire. This is a prime example of the cause of the problem not originating in the affected organ. The cumulative taxation on her foundational kidney energy from the internal and external stress of her competitive childhood through college years essentially exhausted her. The intense work and pressures of graduate school added to this exhaustion, and her kidney fire was no longer able to perform its function as pilot light for her digestive process. Ice cold drinks and cold food further taxed her stomach fire over the years until it caused her digestion to cease. The treatment strategy was first to strengthen the kidney fire, then return it to the stomach. This was accomplished using the appropriate acupuncture points and channels to support these principles. Elimination of cold drinks and food was an important part of the process.

CASE STUDY

Another patient was a 21-year-old female college student. Three months prior to seeking treatment with me, she had fractured a bone in her foot while running stadium stairs. During that time, according to the X-ray, her bone had not healed at all and she was in constant pain. This condition is called "nonunion of fracture" in modern medicine. She wanted to try acupuncture to see if it would help her foot start to heal.

While her orthopedist was deciding whether to consider surgery, we had ten days to fit in three treatments. After each treatment, her pain diminished. The follow-up X-ray showed union of the bone and advanced healing of the fracture. She was very pleased that surgery would not be required.

The treatment strategy in her case was to return Wei Chi to the site of the fracture to perform repair. I accomplished this by using the Divergent Channels which connect Wei Chi to the bone level. Only five needles were required for her treatment. The likely underlying cause preventing proper healing was the use of ice on her foot to reduce swelling after the injury. Ice drives Wei Chi away from an injury site resulting in impaired healing and/ or future arthritis.

CASE STUDY

My final example of successful treatment with acupuncture is a 77-year-old man with recurring lower back and leg pain due to spinal deterioration that was not helped by surgery. He was taking a cocktail of pharmaceuticals for various health issues plus two different pain relievers, including an opiate, for his back pain. His orthopedist suggested he try acupuncture. Because his condition was long-term and because opiates and surgery had already been tried, I was frank with him and said it would likely be a slow process toward relief. I suggested he schedule two treatments per week for three months. He followed through with this plan and, working with his doctor, was able to slowly cut back on his pain medications with no increase in symptoms. After three months we reduced his treatment regimen to once a week. After five months, he had stopped all opiate use, and was taking primarily over-the-counter anti-inflammatories as needed.

He continued to come in every two weeks, then three, then once a month for support. In three years, his episodes of increased pain were easily managed with only over-the-counter medication.

This represents another good example of treating the underlying cause of a problem. The treatment strategy was to increase production of Ying Chi (fuel energy) at the level of his stomach and digestion. I accomplished this by needling points on his stomach and kidney channels to increase digestive strength so he could derive more energy from his food. This patient led a very busy and meaningful life which consumed a great amount of energy. By treating his digestive function, he felt better overall and had more active Yang energy to strengthen his lower back and reduce his pain.

IN SUMMARY:

- Acupuncture works.
- Chinese medical theory is very different from modern medicine, but describes exactly the same concepts.
- We are indoctrinated into believing a quantitative, scientific view of our bodies and health. It is often the only model we have known. It is challenging to accept that a completely different model, one based on qualitative assessment, can be valid.
- The qualitative science of Chinese medicine uses organizational models that describe the essential nature of our body, mind, and spirit—our complete selves.

- Qualitative case studies, used as empirical data, are the primary evidence that acupuncture works. Sometimes definitive material changes like improved blood tests or X-ray images validate the results of acupuncture.

CHAPTER 4

How Does Acupuncture Work?

How does acupuncture work? How does inserting needles into invisible points on the body change pain, disease, and dysfunction? If there is no medication in or on the needle, and treatments are not supplemented with orally administered drugs or vitamins, how does acupuncture help?

Acupuncture appears to be an exotic, radically different approach to treating illness. We always want to know how things work. It is part of our inquisitive nature as human beings. I would love to be able to say, "I put needle A into point B and it corrects condition C." But I cannot. Acupuncture is not a connect-the-dots-with-a-prescribed-process kind of medicine.

As stated in the introduction, there is no current information model that gives us the words to describe how acupuncture works. The science of Chinese medical theory can only be understood on its own terms through its own organizational models and concepts. Our Energetic System cannot be explained using modern quantitative science. However, there are some theories from physics that come close to providing logical explanations on how it may work. I will cover those topics later in the chapter.

When I sit down with my patients for the first time, I briefly review the following organizational models of Chinese medical theory to help them understand the diagnostic process:

Energy
Yin and Yang
Five Phases
Energy Channels
Three Burners
Pulse and Tongue Diagnosis

Their direct experience during and following treatments reinforces these concepts.

Energy
Acupuncture is a type of Holistic Medicine. A "holistic" approach takes into account all aspects of the whole patient—physical, emotional, mental, spiritual, environmental, etc., as opposed to focusing on an individual part, symptom, system or disease.

Acupuncture may also be referred to as Complementary and Alternative Medicine (CAM). Yes, acupuncture can be complementary to modern medicine, but it is also a complete healthcare model in itself. It should be the first choice of treatment for all medical conditions that are not imminently life-threatening.

Acupuncture is Energetic Medicine. This means that it works with the energies of our bodies that direct structure, function, and protection. It employs energy therapy instead of chemical and/or surgical therapies. Other energetic modalities include Reiki, Homeopathy, Ayurveda, and Bioresonance therapies.

Energy is defined in a lot of ways. We commonly refer to it in the context of commodities traded to supply power to our homes and cars: gas, electric, nuclear, wind, or solar energy. We also use it to describe our physical capacity for doing work, "She has a lot of energy today." Or conversely, "I am so tired after that workout, I have no energy left."

The first law of thermodynamics teaches us that energy is a conserved quantity that can be neither created nor destroyed, only transferred from one form to another. The energy we most commonly consider in our bodies is that generated by the chemical breakdown of food through digestion, and oxygen absorbed through respiration. This energy is measured in joules or calories. In Chinese medical theory, calories from food and oxygen are only one variety of human energy, Ying Chi (fuel energy). There are several others that I will explain throughout this book. For example, we have all heard statements like, "She really has a lot of positive energy," and "there is a lot of negative energy in the room today." These statements don't refer to calories of energy, but to a spiritual or emotional energy that can't be measured. In Chinese medicine this is called our Shen (spiritual energy).

Remember the moving leaf and wind metaphor from the last chapter? Our energetic system is the wind—that unseeable, immeasurable force within us that animates our life. Without energy we would not be living beings.

From a modern medical perspective, we believe that the smartest physical system in the body is the nervous system. The brain controls everything, but what controls the neurons that cause the brain to function? How does each cell in our central nervous system know what to do? The answer—Energy! It is our operating system. Our brain "application" cannot function without its "operating system."

Energy circulates in channels in the body. These channels, or rivers of energy, are commonly called meridians in the English language. "Meridian" is an inaccurate term that originated with early western explorers to China who arrived by sea. As sailors, they saw the lines depicting the energy channels on acupuncture charts and referred to them as meridian lines, like those from their nautical charts. Unlike the arbitrarily-assigned longitudinal lines on a map, the lines of acupuncture charts represent trajectories of dynamic action or movement throughout the body. Therefore, I refer to them as energy channels.

Before we look at energy channels in greater depth, I need to provide more context. The channels are only one aspect of our organ systems, so we will first examine the organizational models that describe these systems. The models describe, first and foremost, how nature works, so it is impossible to discuss them without reference to these actions. I will, however, focus more on their application to human health.

Yin and Yang

The symbol of Yin and Yang has very deep-reaching meaning. (See Fig. 9.) It describes how everything in nature is interrelated. There cannot be Yin separate from Yang, and Yang contains a little drop of Yin. It also explains that the energy of heaven (Yang) and the energy of earth (Yin) meet to form the unique biosphere of our planet. The space where heaven and earth meet is where we humans exist alongside many other wildly-varied life-forms.

In human health, Yin and Yang are simply another description of our anatomy and physiology. They describe form and function. Yin is form—the physical organs that may be observed with an MRI or surgery. Yang is the function the organ performs, like the filtration of waste by your kidneys or the digestion of food by your stomach.

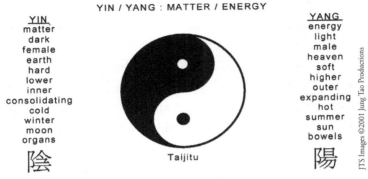

YIN / YANG : MATTER / ENERGY

YIN	YANG
matter	energy
dark	light
female	male
earth	heaven
hard	soft
lower	higher
inner	outer
consolidating	expanding
cold	hot
winter	summer
moon	sun
organs	bowels

Taijitu

陰   陽

JTS Images ©2001 Jung Tao Productions

Fig. 9 Yin/Yang Symbol and Associations

The concept of Yin and Yang is more than simply form and function though. For example, the orifices in our heads (eyes, nose, mouth, and ears) are the portals of our senses through which we perceive the world. Other than their being on or off, we do not quantify them with measurement. We do not say, "John can only smell 30 units of olfaction instead of 90." Or, "Betty saw 1,000,000 pixels of trees today." Our perceptions, therefore, are more Yang—immaterial if you will—not quantifiable. They are, however, dependent on our Yin structures to become Yang perceptions.

Likewise, our emotions (anger, joy, worry, sadness, fear) are immaterial. There are not 100 quivers of fear or 25 jumps of joy. We know that we feel the Yang response of emotion, but material science has yet to significantly acknowledge that a Yang emotion can have a disease-inducing effect on Yin structure.

The Yin-Yang symbol represents the two as inseparable. Everything in existence is made up of matter and energy. Some things tend toward Yin, like a rock, and some toward Yang, like air. But the rock can emit radiation which is Yang energy; and the air contains physical (Yin) molecules like oxygen and carbon dioxide. Similarly, there is not a Yang thought without a Yin body to produce it.

Humans inherently tend to be imbalanced toward Yang. Our huge brain requires a vast amount of material energy (nutrients via the blood) to produce Yang thoughts. To a minor degree, our active Yang brains keep us in a slightly Yin-deficient state. Thoughts allow us to explore with our imagination and be physically more active than our survival requires. Modern Western culture, with its emphasis on success and achievement and constant stimulation, adds to our Yang-ness. Stillness, contemplation, rest, and receptiveness are Yin states, and are necessary to replenish our Yin material.

A very stark example of Yin-Yang in humans is abuse of the drug, methamphetamine. Before-and-after photos of the afflicted tell the story. Before drug use, meth users show round, fleshy faces and bodies. Photos of these same people taken several months after meth use show them with gaunt faces and skinny bodies. Their Yin flesh has been consumed, melted away by the hot Yang drug.

Yin and Yang are considered diagnostically with concepts such as the internal balance of hot and cold. The Yin channels traverse the dark, front side of the body; and the Yang channels traverse the light, back side of the body.

The Five Phases: Five Organ Systems

There are five aspects of nature commonly referred to in the West as the Five Elements (Wood, Fire, Earth, Metal, and Water). Like the word "meridian," *element* is an imprecise choice of words since its connotation is that of an ingredient or singular part. I prefer the term *phase* as defined in modern physics as matter's ability to exist in different states. Take, for example, water. Depending on its molecular arrangement, it can be either gaseous, solid or liquid in form, with each phase having its own individual properties. In Chinese medicine, these five elements or phases relate to the five organ systems in the human body.

This description is more in-line with the idea of nature and the concept of the organ system in Chinese medicine. Each component of nature and each organ system is comprised of a spectrum of attributes, different states of matter and energy, and therefore, different phases. In human health, this correlates to our physical body parts, our senses of perception, our emotions, and our spiritual aspect. For this reason, I will refer to our organ systems as the Five Phases.

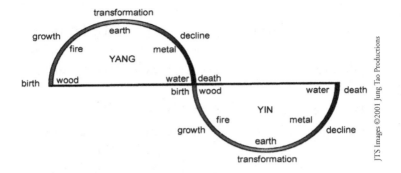

Fig. 10 Five Phases: Time

Acupuncturists use the Five Phases model as one lens through which they evaluate the current state of their patient. Clues such as skin color, sleep quality, emotional struggles, or bowel activity all point to which phase/organ system(s) is struggling. That system's channel can then be used to correct the imbalance therapeutically to restore health. Acupuncture points along the channel are chosen for the unique effect they have on that organ system, and their relationship to the entire system of the patient.

There are several configurations of Five Phases that describe general relationships in nature. The first arrangement describes the cycle of life. (See Fig. 10.) The season of Wood is spring, or the time of birth in nature. The season of Fire is summer, or the season of growth. Between seasons there is a period of transformation which is Earth. After summer comes fall, or Metal, the season of decline. And winter, or Water, closes out the yearly cycle as the season of death. The cycle repeats as spring follows winter.

Our lives mimic this cycle of nature. A patient's location (age) on the continuum of the birth/death spectrum is a factor considered in diagnosis. Likewise, the season of the year when a treatment takes place is also taken into account. Certain illnesses prevail during certain seasons, like flu (wind/cold) in winter. In my practice, I encourage healthy patients to come in for seasonal tune-ups to help them sync with the greater climate as it transitions to the next season. This helps them respond to environmental conditions more favorably and reduces their chance of becoming sick.

Another configuration of the Five Phases describes how the various aspects of nature interrelate, and therefore, how our organ systems interrelate. The Sheng-Ko cycle describes creation/generation (Sheng) and control (Ko).

In Fig. 11, we see that the phases are all connected. The clockwise progression shows the Sheng, or generating cycle. Wood (liver/gallbladder) is the mother of Fire (heart/small intestine). It gives fire energy to fuel function. Fire (heart/small intestine) is the mother of Earth (spleen/stomach). Earth is the mother of Metal (lung/large intestine). Metal is the mother of Water (kidney/bladder) which is the mother of Wood.

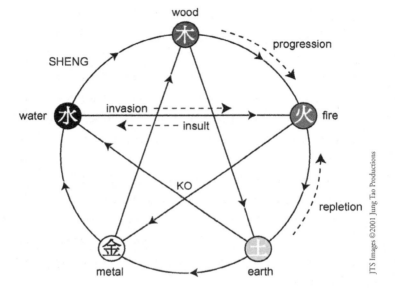

Fig. 11 Five Phases: Sheng-Ko

The star formation represents the Ko, or controlling relationships, between the phases. If, for example, Earth gets its generating energy from Fire, then Wood controls, regulates, or modulates Earth. This is nature's system of checks and balances, preventing life from spinning out of control. This is similar to homeostasis or autoregulation in modern medicine.

Phase Association is the organizational model in which all attributes of the human being are categorized into organ systems. The way an organ is perceived in traditional Chinese medicine is quite different from anatomy and physiology portrayed by modern medicine.

For example, the Water phase includes: teeth and bones; the kidney and urinary bladder; reproductive, central nervous and endocrine systems; cerebrospinal and synovial fluids; ears and sense of hearing; emotions of fear and paranoia; the spiritual aspect of Zhi (will and volition); and all of the tissues and structures traversed by the kidney and bladder channels. (See Table 1.)

Phase associations give us a comprehensive view of ourselves. The Water phase, for example, includes both the kidney organ and fear. When one is addressed in treatment, the other is affected. Assessment through the Five Phases helps us understand how seemingly-unconnected problems in our life or body are actually related. During a diagnosis, the Five Phases come into play in different configurations and different ways. When the source of an illness is considered, the Sheng-Ko model is useful. For example, asthma is a condition that exhibits symptoms of breathing difficulty in the lungs. From the Sheng-Ko cycle there are several possibilities for the source of asthma. It could be due to weakness in the lung (Metal), or it could be due to the spleen/stomach (Earth) being weak and being unable to send generating energy to the lung. Asthma could also originate in the bladder/kidney (Water). This is symbolic of a child weakening its mother by draining her energy. These are just a few of the possible origins from which a diagnosis and treatment for asthma might evolve.

	WOOD	**FIRE**
YIN ORGAN	liver	heart-emperial xin bao-ministerial
YANG BOWEL	gall bladder	small intestine san jiao
BODY TISSUES	muscles-sinews motor neurons	blood vessels
FLOWERING	eyes-nails	tongue
SECRETION	tears	perspiration
SENSE	vision	speech
JING SHEN	hun (creativity)	shen (spirit)
EMOTIONAL	creativity-judgment anger	consciousness unconsciousness
CLIMATE	wind	heat
SEASON	spring	summer
COLOR	green	red
DIRECTION	east	south
SAPOR	sour	bitter
SMELL	rancid-sour	scorched
VOICE	screaming-yelling shouting	laughing
FUNCTIONS	wei qi production storage of blood	metabolism blood circulation
DEVELOPMENTAL	birth	growth
MUSICAL SOUND	jiao	zheng

Table 1 Phase Association chart

EARTH	METAL	WATER
spleen	lung	kidney
stomach	large intestine	bladder
dermis	epidermis-sensory nerves body hair-pores	bone-teeth-CNS head and pubic hair
mouth-lips-gums	nose	ears
saliva	mucous	urine
taste	smell	hearing
yi (self awareness)	po (sensitivity)	zhi (will)
thought-intellect obsession-worry	sensitivity hypersensitivity-grief	will-volition fear
humidity	dryness	cold
seasonal transitions	fall	winter
yellow	clear	black
center	west	north
sweet	pungent	salty
aromatic-perfumed	raw meat	putrid
singing	weeping	moaning-sighing
distribution of sapors and nutritional liquids	begins classical order	source organ storage of yuan qi
transformation	decline	death
gong	shang	yu

The origin of a health problem isn't determined solely by signs and symptoms, but also by evaluating energetic pulses taken at the wrists where the different organs and their relationships present themselves.

The Energetic Channels

Eight Extraordinary, Primary, Sinew, Luo, and Divergent Channels

Each yin organ and yang bowel has an energy channel with acupuncture points along it as part of its system. The channels offer another diagnostic model, as well as being the interface where your acupuncturist can use needles to treat dysfunction.

There are five classes of energy channels. (See Fig. 12.) Three of the five energy channels must be functioning for a human to be alive. In order to survive in a hostile world, the other two arise on demand to protect us from acute or chronic external attacks.

Eight Extraordinary Channels

The Eight Extraordinary Channels are the realm of our Yuan Chi (ancestral energy). This is similar to modern science's concept of DNA. The Eight Extraordinary Channels keep our blueprint in circulation, telling every cell in our body how to organize itself and how to function.

The Eight Extraordinary Channels are the framework for our anatomy, physiology, and psychology. They explain not only our inherited traits, but also how the influence of life and the environment affect genetic expression, or epigenetics.

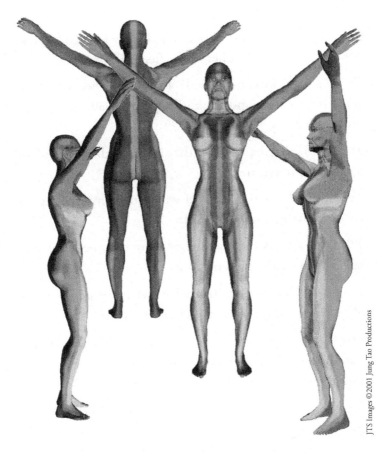

JTS Images ©2001 Jung Tao Productions

Fig. 12 Human figure showing all channels throughout the body

Included in the Eight Extraordinary Channels:

Chong Mai is the first channel to form when egg and sperm unite. It distributes our life destiny, plan or curriculum.

Ren Mai is the channel of bonding, ideally formed by close connection to our mother in the first three years of life.

Du Mai is the channel of independence. It becomes fully active when we stand up and begin to walk away from our mother.

Yin Wei Mai is the channel that is a recording of our life up to the present moment.

Yang Wei Mai is the channel where the physical experiences of the past are recorded.

Yin Qiao Mai is the channel of whom we perceive ourselves to be at the present time.

Yang Qiao Mai is the channel of what we perceive our place in the world to be at the present time.

Dai Mai is the channel which is a receptacle that houses the challenges of life's curriculum which cannot be resolved and must be passed on to future generations.

My teacher, Ann Cecil-Sterman, describes these channels in her outstanding instructional book, *Advanced Acupuncture: A Clinic Manual*:

"The Eight Extras are conduits of constitutional Chi

(Yuan Qi). Yuan Qi contains our ancestral inheritance, our nature. The Eight Extras therefore govern the creation of form. The first Eight Extra, the Chong, is the blueprint; it's like a set of construction drawings. The Ren Channel is like a warehouse that stores or provides the materials (Yin) for the building. The Du is like the construction crew that provides the energy (Yang) to build the building, according to the blueprint stored in the Chong. The building performs its function in space, aging and changing through time. The Wei Channels govern the assimilation of these changes. The Qiao Channels reflect the present.

The building inspector can give a report on the building's current status (Yin Qiao) and also how the building now fits into the streetscape, its current context (Yang Qiao). The Wei Channels record the way in which the building came to be the way it is. The building inspector might document the changes the building has undergone in its long history (Yin Wei Mai) and make predictions about how it will age in the future, and what the building will need (Yang Wei Mai). The Dai Mai would function as storage, sanitation, and a clearing house for trash."

Therapeutically, the Eight Extraordinary Channels are used to address problems existing since childhood and other long-standing problems.

The Three Burners

The Three Burners are not channels, but the source of the energies that circulate in the next two classes of channels. (See Fig. 13.) The Eight Extraordinary Channels erect and direct our three-level energy production plant (Three Burners) where we turn food and oxygen into fuel and defensive energy.

The Middle Burner is represented in the stomach, spleen, and small intestine. Food, the energy of the earth, arrives in the middle burner where it is heated and cooked to release its energy and nutrients.

The Upper Burner is represented in the lung and heart. Here, the food energy from the middle burner is combined with the energy of heaven/oxygen to make our Ying Chi (fuel energy). The heart then propels fuel-rich blood into circulation through the blood vessels, and the energy of the primary channels leads it where it needs to go. In a healthy state and with proper diet, we produce fuel energy in excess which we store to conserve our Yuan Chi for times of illness or famine.

The Lower Burner is represented in the large intestine, liver, gallbladder, kidney, and bladder. This is our detoxification center where waste products generated by burning fuel energy are eliminated.

During diagnosis, the Three Burners organizational model helps the acupuncturist identify the location of dysfunction and how it relates to the entire system. From the case studies in Chapter 2 we saw how stomach dysfunction (Middle Burner) had its origin in kidney fire (Lower Burner).

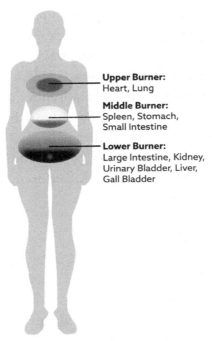

Upper Burner:
Heart, Lung

Middle Burner:
Spleen, Stomach,
Small Intestine

Lower Burner:
Large Intestine, Kidney,
Urinary Bladder, Liver,
Gall Bladder

Fig. 13 The Three Burners

Primary Channels

Primary Channels are the realm of our Ying Chi (fuel energy). Energy produced by the Three Burners is distributed from our organs to the cells in our body via the Primary Channels. They are the delivery network, the highway system of the body, and should be open and unimpeded so our internal goods and services can reach their destination as easily and efficiently as possible.

The Primary Channels carry the names of their solid organ or hollow bowel origin. They flow from these places, traversing the trunk to the limbs, terminating in the tips of our fingers and toes. Their trajectories are represented by lines on the acupuncture charts. Their names are Lung, Large Intestine, Stomach, Spleen, Heart, Small Intestine, Bladder, Kidney, Pericardium, Triple Heater, Gallbladder, and Liver. The Primary Channels connect the internal organs to each other and describe the day-to-day flow of life. Therapeutically, they correct disrupted internal connections and help restore normal function to build and maintain our resources.

Sinew Channels

The Sinew Channels are located in our skin, muscles, tendons and ligaments. This is the third channel system that must function for us to live.

In order to protect our internal parts from attack by outside forces, we must have an initial defense system. The Sinew Channels, the conduits of our Wei Chi (defensive energy), reside at the surface to protect us from external attacks. Wei Chi also circulates deeply, more internally, where it is needed to repair damaged or worn parts. It is constantly on the move, cycling from inside to outside, scouting for enemy attacks and damaged infrastructure. Wei Chi is a hot, vaporous energy that when summoned creates the hallmarks of what modern medicine calls inflammation: heat, swelling, and pain. Wei Chi also moves our limbs, making escape part of our defense.

The Sinew Channels not only protect us in the physical sense, as in modern germ theory, but also offer emotional protection, forming an external barrier against the psychological assaults of life.

Chinese medicine recognizes the origin of disease as being either external or internal. Disease of external origin describes infection from physical and emotional pathogens that have penetrated the Sinew Channels from outside the body. Disease of internal origin describes health problems, including physical illness, caused by our internal thoughts and feelings. As either external- or internal-origin diseases heal, they pass out of the body through the Sinew Channels—permanently expelled from our body and mind.

Luo and Divergent Channels

Luo and Divergent Channels are our survival mechanisms. They are secondary protection channels that arise on demand to shunt assaults that are strong enough to penetrate the Sinew Channels into a holding area away from the Primary Channels. This function is crucial to survival because any pathology, emotional or physiological, left unchecked in the Primary Channels can progress all the way to an organ. There it can quickly become life-threatening. The Luo and Divergent channels act as jails to protect our organs from these pathologies. The Luos use the limbs and Divergents use the major joints as way stations.

The Luo Channels hold unwelcome energy hostage in our limbs. Visible blood vessels, like spider and varicose veins, are Luo Vessels. There the body uses stagnant blood as its medium of captivity. Since, in Chinese medicine, "the heart is the blood is the emotions," emotional pathology is generally held captive in these channels. By locking down pathology in the limbs, the body creates small aches and pains or impedes mobility, but our organs remain safe from harm. This is called Disease Nemesis Theory. Treating emotional issues is a particular strength of the Luos.

Divergent Channels store unwelcome energy in our major joints (knees, shoulders, hips), or in our spine, teeth, or brain. The dense tissue (cartilage and marrow) in these areas lock down pathology. Again, our bodies will create small problems like back, knee, or shoulder pain in order to protect the major organs from more serious illnesses. Pathology held in the Divergents taxes our resources and leads to degeneration of the joints, spine, teeth and brain. The Divergent Channels are the system used to describe and treat chronic degenerative diseases.

These five classes of channels function together orchestrating and reacting to life. When an imbalance, dysfunction, or disease presents itself, the channel system is engaged therapeutically to return us to a state of health. The acupuncturist will choose the most appropriate energy channel and acupuncture points based on presenting signs and symptoms.

- The Eight Extraordinary Channels are used to address problems present since childhood or very old problems.
- The Principal Channels are used to strengthen day-to-day function.
- The Sinew Channels are used to treat acute illness or injury.
- The Luo Channels are used to help with emotional issues or older injuries of the limbs.
- The Divergent Channels are used to treat chronic degenerative and autoimmune illnesses.

Pulses

In Chinese medical diagnosis, pulse assessment yields an enormous amount of information about the body's internal condition, or *milieu interieur*. Imagine the acupuncturist as a diagnostic device. The pulses are the interface through which they gain insight into the patient's current internal status.

Energetic pulses are felt at the wrist on the radial artery, the same place where modern medical doctors take your pulse. These pulses carry much more information than just the number of heartbeats per minute. There are three pulse positions on each wrist. Each position represents one of the organ systems.

The pulse locations on the right wrist indicate lung/ large intestine, spleen/stomach, and pericardium/Triple Heater organs. These are the energy pulses representing Yang, active energy. (See Fig. 14a.)

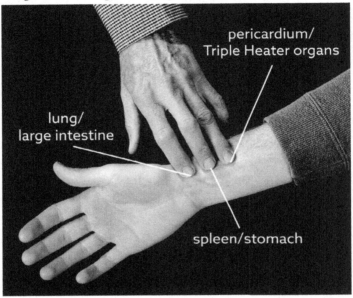

Fig. 14a Pulse Positions, right hand

The pulse locations on the left wrist indicate heart/ small intestine, liver/gallbladder, and kidney/bladder organs. These are the blood pulses representing Yin, material energy. (See Fig. 14b.)

You may be wondering what can be felt in a pulse other than heartbeats-per-minute. It is estimated that there are approximately 100,000 kilometers, or 62,000 miles of blood vessels running through your body. Quite a stunning figure really. From the pump-and-pipes perspective of modern science, the heart is the pump that pushes blood through and around this giant network of vessels, or pipes.

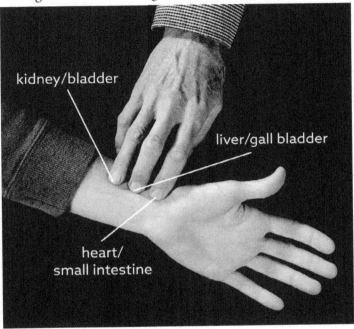

kidney/bladder

liver/gall bladder

heart/
small intestine

Fig. 14b Pulse Positions, left hand

Chinese medical theory, however, states that the heart launches blood into circulation in the blood vessels, and that energy circulating in the energetic channels leads it around the body. The Yin/Yang concept describes the material, Yin (blood), as animated by the immaterial, Yang (energy). Yang energy creates a magnetic field which attracts and moves Yin iron in the blood, pulling it along.

Blood circulation can be compared to the flow of water in a river. Some may imagine that water wells up from a source and is pushed downhill from a force behind it. Instead, invisible, immaterial Yang energy (gravity) is pulling the visible, material Yin substance (water) downward. Stand beside a creek or river. Try to view its flow from that perspective, and you will get a sense of how blood moves through the body.

Within the pulses rides a great deal of information, not unlike the signal transmissions of our modern technological communication devices. Just as telephone, television, and internet signals travel in the same cable, parallel signals transmitted in our pulses communicate blood volume, fluid status, immune function and more.

Specific information examined by your acupuncturist at each pulse position includes height, length, depth, width, speed (in beats-per-respiratory-cycle), and quality or feel at each location. The list of qualities contain descriptions like tight, slippery, choppy, or leathery. Each quality exposes a state of the internal climate such as cold, hot, damp, or stagnant.

Using Dynamic-Pulse-Reading technique, communication between the organ systems is assessed. This provides information about the internal state of autoregulation, or the Sheng-Ko cycle of generation and control.

Finally, as your acupuncturist's fingers press more

deeply into your wrist, an exploration of the entire channel system is possible. First, at the surface, are the Sinew Channels, the realm of Wei Chi. Next, at the moderate level, are the Principal Channels where our Ying Chi circulates. Deep at the level of the bone lie the Eight Extraordinary Channels, where Yuan Chi lives. The Divergent Channels also appear at the deep level. There are no pulses for the Luo Channels since they are visible to the eye on the surface of the skin.

It takes years of experience, observation and study as a practitioner to comprehend the myriad of possibilities that can be sensed in the pulses. There are Chinese medical physicians who, after listening carefully to a patient's pulses, can describe conditions that existed decades earlier. My patients often express surprise when I diagnose a tight neck or diet containing cold foods and drink simply from listening to their pulses. The energetic pulses convey a vast amount of information about their lives and health. As I have developed more sensitive pulse-listening skills over the years, I've been able to help my patients through their treatments in a more meaningful way. This is the richest source of knowledge in the array of diagnostic models available to me.

Tongue Examination
Many patients, especially children, find it entertaining that I examine their tongues. But our tongues are another

source of diagnostic information. Like our pulses, our tongues are indicators of health. (See Fig. 15.)

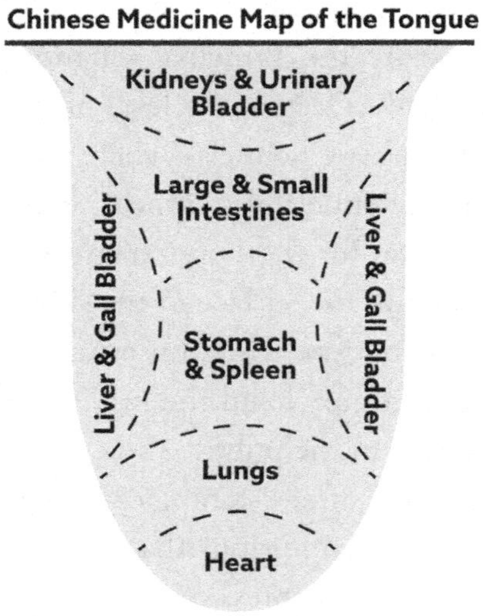

Chinese Medicine Map of the Tongue

Fig. 15 Tongue Examination

So what does the tongue reveal about a patient's health? First, color indicates the temperature of their internal climate. Red is hot. Pale is cold. Next, the coating tells me about the state of fluids in the system. Thin and white is normal. Thick and yellow signifies internal dampness and heat. Size and shape indicate status of organ function. A swollen tongue with wavy edges indicates worry which affects the spleen/stomach organs. The location of features like bumps, bare patches, cracks, and sores offers hints to which organ is affected.

If a tongue is red, thin, cracked, and uncoated, this

tells me there is internal heat and inflammation. Cracking would indicate long-term dehydration or stress which has diminished the kidney Yin, creating a hot internal climate. It could also mean that the patient's diet is high in sugar and other immune-stimulating foods. Thinness of the tongue and lack of coating means the condition has likely existed for a long time, and that heat has evaporated body fluids like hormones and spinal fluid.

In summary, these organizational models of Chinese medical theory are based on a structured set of principles, and while they are different from the models of modern medical science, they are no less stringent or comprehensive. The practice of Chinese medicine over millennia is a testament to its validity and effectiveness.

How Does Acupuncture Work?

No one knows the mechanical science behind what makes acupuncture work, but I have witnessed and experienced its effectiveness time and again. Is there a modern scientific explanation for what happens when a needle is placed into an acupuncture point?

Modern medicine categorizes human beings predominantly through the lenses of biology and biochemistry. Biology includes anatomy, the branch of biology concerned with the study of the structure of organisms and their parts. Surgery is the tool most often employed for health problems diagnosed as mechanical in origin.

Biology also includes physiology, the scientific study of the functions and mechanisms which work within a living system. It focuses on how organisms, organ systems, organs, cells, and biomolecules carry out the chemical and physical functions that exist in a living system. This includes biochemical functions. Modern medicine's approach to disease management and treatment relies on chemical intervention to modify biochemical functions.

Energetic medicine is not included in either of the sciences just mentioned, but there is another modern science that addresses concepts of energy—quantum physics.

My first acupuncture teacher, the late Dr. Sean Marshall, was, among other things, very interested in quantum physics. He posited that this particular area of science might provide some insight as to how acupuncture works. I will expand on some of his original ideas here.

Theories borrowed from classical and quantum physics, the study of matter and energy (Yin and Yang), come the closest to describing how and from where acupuncture may derive its healing power and effectiveness.

Most people understand classic physics from what they learned in high school—basic concepts of gravity, inertia, mass, force, momentum, etc. The laws of physics govern the macroscopic world. We see an apple fall to the ground from a tree and understand the earth's gravitational force on an object.

In a nutshell, quantum physics is the study of invisible matter—particles, subatomic particles, atoms, electrons, light waves, etc.—the building blocks that make up everything around us, including us. What makes quantum physics so unusual is that the laws of "normal" physics no longer apply in the realm of the super small. Albert Einstein and Niels Bohr were among the first to figure this out.

The first theoretical mechanism of acupuncture is derived from classical physics' concept of electromagnetic fields. Electromagnetism creates fields of energy that radiate outward from a source and interact with other such fields. It has been observed that if there is interference in such a field at any point, there is instantaneous, simultaneous change in the entire field. It is possible that the level of energy that comprises our energetic system is electromagnetism.

Now, let's imagine that each of the five organ systems represents the source of an electromagnetic field. There are five fields that overlap and interact. Putting a metal needle into a point anywhere in one field would cause instantaneous, simultaneous change in all five fields. Our energy underlies all form and function; therefore, when a needle realigns these fields it necessarily changes our physical and chemical states of being and, therefore, our health. (See Fig. 16.)

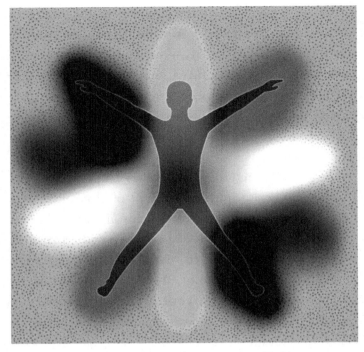

Fig. 16 Our Five Electromagnetic Fields

The second theoretical mechanism of acupuncture comes from quantum physics. It is possible that a needle engages our energy channels as a connection to an enormous storehouse of potential energy within the body to stimulate or release a new ability to function at a higher level. What is this enormous storehouse of energy and where is it located? Remember Einstein's famous mathematical equation, $E=mc^2$? This equation is simply another way to describe the ancient Chinese symbol of Yin and Yang, or matter and energy.

If you were like me in high school, the math and concepts behind Einstein's equation describing energy's relation to mass and the speed of light were difficult to comprehend. It was explained to me again much later in life by Dr. Marshall in the context of its relationship to the human body. I break it down here:

E = Energy
m = Mass (weight minus the effect of gravity)
c = Speed of Light

So, $E=mc^2$ states that Energy is equal to Mass multiplied by the Speed of Light squared.

The essence of this equation is that a tiny amount of material (mass) contains a huge amount of potential energy (E). Start with c, the speed of light. This is a really big number. Rounded off it is 300,000,000 (three hundred million) meters per second. Now multiply that by itself and you have c^2—a really, really big number. Multiply c^2 by the mass of an object, and you have calculated its potential energy.

To give this some real-world perspective, consider the average human being weighing 154 pounds has a mass of 70 kg. Plug that number into Einstein's equation, E = 70 x 300,000,000 x 300,000,000, and you begin to get an idea of the extraordinary potential energy one person contains.

So what can a person do with all that potential energy? Through some more complicated math, we can figure out the power of this energy to do work. The resulting potential energy of a 154-pound person can run a 100-watt light bulb for about two billion years! Humans are electrifying!

I surmise that acupuncture somehow taps into this enormous well of potential energy as its mechanism of action. Just a tiny drop of this energy brought back into circulation in our body could literally jumpstart healing and growth.

I like this theory, but have no idea how sticking a needle into an acupuncture point causes this potentiation. However, experience shows me that *something* is happening. It is a mystery, quite possibly unknowable via traditional quantitative science, but this theory may one day be substantiated through further study of elementary particles like the Higgs boson, also known as the God particle, discovered as recently as 2013.

These are very interesting theories to contemplate. We don't yet fully understand how acupuncture works using modern scientific explanation, but it isn't necessary to know how it works for it to work. Modern scientific theories, in all branches of study, change and shift over time as new discoveries are made. Perhaps in the years to come, we will break new ground in science as research continues to develop as-yet-uninvented technologies that may offer more tangible, concrete explanations for how acupuncture works.

IN SUMMARY:

- From my own experience undergoing acupuncture, and from administering over 15,000 acupuncture treatments, I can say definitively, it does work.
- Acupuncture causes some materially-unknown mechanism in our body to induce healing and improve health.
- The best way to understand how acupuncture works is to experience it yourself.
- Familiarity with the organizational models of Chinese medicine can help you understand the terminology your acupuncturist uses and the organization of his or her diagnostic process.
- Modern quantitative science may one day uncover and describe in concrete terms how acupuncture taps into our potential energy, be it physical, emotional, or spiritual, to fuel healing and personal growth.

CHAPTER 5

What Health Problems Does Acupuncture Treat?

We live in the age of specialization and sub-specialization by physicians in modern medical disease management. Family practice doctors and internists examine patients generally, then often refer them to specialists. It is hard to imagine a single medical model that can diagnose and treat the entire spectrum of mental and physical health. Acupuncture, with its holistic approach, is perfect for addressing a wide range of issues.

The channel system, in particular, describes how genetics (Eight Extraordinary Channels), day-to-day energy production and distribution (Primary Channels), immune function (Sinew Channels), and emotional and physical difficulties (Luo and Divergent Channels) influence us. These channels also allow acupuncturists to therapeutically influence all locations, depths, functions, and dysfunctions of the human being—emotional and physical.

With a few exceptions, acupuncture should be the first stop in healthcare, not the last resort. Acupuncture is the medical intervention with the greatest potential for healing and the least risk of damage. It is the simplest approach possible since it enables self-healing and introduces no chemical substances into the body. Chinese medical theory also offers meaningful, time-tested information on the effects of diet on health.

Many years ago I listened to an interview with a Dutch medical doctor. His objective was to avoid pharmaceutical treatment for his patients as long as possible. He tried an array of milder therapies before resorting to any drug or surgery. Alternative options he considered included psychoanalysis and counseling, nutritional advice and meditation, yoga and Tai Chi, massage therapy and prayer, and energetic treatments like acupuncture, Healing Touch, Reiki, Ayurvedic medicine, spiritual healing and herbal remedies.

Be wary of modern medicine's all-too-common approach to jump straight to drugs or surgery. These are very powerful interventions. They can be extremely valuable in some cases, but should only be considered if there is no other way. It's a little like using a sledgehammer to hang a picture when a tack hammer will do. The likelihood of collateral damage is much higher, and in the case of surgery it is impossible to reset to the beginning if things don't work out the first time.

The list of health issues and diseases I have treated with acupuncture is long. Patients have come to me with anxiety, depression, back pain, headaches, gastroparesis, broken bones, macular degeneration, IBS, constipation, gallbladder attacks, atrial fibrillation, neuropathy, varicose veins, chronic viral infections, diabetes, sports injuries, and more. Referrals from an oncologist have allowed me to see how acupuncture has helped cancer patients negotiate the rigors of chemotherapy. I have shepherded one of my patients, who is highly allergic to Novocaine, through several dental fillings, a root canal, and a tooth extraction using only acupuncture for pain control. However, the main premise of treatment using Chinese medicine is to reestablish health, not treat disease. In the presence of health, disease cannot exist.

An unfortunate side effect of modern medicine is that we only go to the doctor when there is something wrong. In the absence of illness, modern medicine's disease management model has little to offer. By the time a disease becomes noticeable, the health train has already been off the tracks for a while. Yes, acupuncture can help when there is something wrong. Equally as important, though, it can treat you when you are healthy. We are incredibly complex beings. Sensitive messages about our state of health are sent through skin color, emotional state, condition of our tongue, body odor, and energetic pulses—all of which can be interpreted in Chinese medicine—allowing us to make subtle adjustments before illness can evolve. Think of it as scheduled maintenance or preventative medicine.

In modern medicine, specialists treat ailments in specific areas of the body. An acupuncturist looks at the whole picture of health in multi-layers and interrelationships. They may treat several different ailments at once. There is always the potential for acupuncture to help any condition.

Modern medicine excels in the treatment of life-threatening trauma and acute medical issues. We are extremely fortunate to have access to the powerful tools that exist in the disease management model. I was grateful to have access to a hospital and well-trained doctors and nurses when I fractured my femur in high school, and again when my heart stopped for a brief time later in life. But there is more to caring for our health than waiting to get sick or injured and then counting on technology to save us. The vast majority of our health problems are not acute or life-threatening. They are chronic and, all too often, progressive. I am awed by how many people put on a happy face, but are secretly living with a significantly painful physical or emotional issue.

In Chinese medical theory it is said that we are given a curriculum in life. The lessons in our curriculum are the struggles, the high and low points, successes and failures, emotional and physical illnesses. They are meant to encourage us to examine our lives and look at its deeper meaning. Our "gut feelings" are the messages we receive from our true selves. However, we are repeatedly told by society, family, religion, etc. that we should be someone else, ignore our feelings and live to the beat of their drum. This diverts us from achieving our fullest potential and living our unique lives.

Helping us return to our destined path in life is one of the most overlooked benefits of acupuncture. Regular treatments that address the myriad of minor flaws and inconsistencies as they arise can enhance overall health and quality of life. We don't have to wait to get sick to go to the doctor. Quarterly, biannual, or yearly tune-ups are a great way to experience the preventative and expansive potentials of acupuncture.

IN SUMMARY:
- Acupuncture offers a general approach to health and can treat a wide range of issues.
- With a few exceptions, acupuncture should be the first stop in healthcare, not the last resort. Going to the doctor when you are sick is a legacy of the disease management model of modern medicine. Acupuncture offers true preventative care with treatments while you are healthy.
- Acupuncture addresses not only health dysfunction, but also presents the possibility to help you live to your fullest potential.

CHAPTER 6

How Many Treatments Will It Take?

We are each unique in our makeup and life experience. This individualizes the healing process for each of us.

The number of acupuncture treatments required for each patient or each ailment varies considerably. Younger patients often respond more quickly than older ones. More recent injuries or problems generally respond sooner than longer-standing ones. There is no reliable way to predict how many treatments you will need for any condition.

When our body, mind, or spirit has been in a state of chronic dysfunction for years or decades, we construct many defensive mechanisms to protect ourselves from further damage. We continue to live because our channels of survival are there absorbing the ongoing assaults of life. We forge ahead, but in a less-than-ideal state of health.

Disease Nemesis Theory states that we create minor problems like limb or joint pain in lieu of major illness. Our Luo and Divergent channels are truly miraculous in this function. Undoing these protective patterns takes time. I have often seen patients improve until they reach a plateau and remain there. Their system becomes incapable of progressing. It remains in protection mode that blocks further improvement.

I have seen movement in many directions from these plateaus. Some patients simply remain there. Others get worse before progressing. Some plateau for years with infrequent supportive treatments, then suddenly experience significant improvement. Finally, there are those who continue to improve slowly over months or years with treatments taken at a frequency they are comfortable with and feel supported by. We are all unique.

Teachers, doctors, attorneys—anyone with emotional stress inherent in their work—find that monthly acupuncture helps them cope better. Patients whose work involves strenuous physical labor, like carpenters or landscapers, find that monthly treatments help ease the physical strain on their bodies. Older patients respond well to weekly or bi-monthly treatments, and are able to experience a higher quality of life with greater vitality and less age-related pain and illness. The patients who come in consistently for a tune-up at supportive intervals generally remain in better overall health, suffering fewer colds and other minor illnesses.

Acupuncture is often sought by patients as a last resort. This is due to the belief that modern medicine is our sole recourse. When drugs, surgery, and/or physical therapy have not helped, and we become desperate for a resolution, only then do we typically become more open to alternatives. We begin to look at treatments we may have considered fringe or questionable. In crisis, we become more willing to step outside of our intellectual comfort zone.

Acupuncture is not magic. It is based on the qualitative scientific concepts of Daoist philosophy. Acupuncturists use the qualitative logic of the organizational models described in this book to diagnose and treat their patients. Acupuncture is a testament to the truth of an ancient Chinese medicine that has been in continuous use for at least 2,000 years.

Dr. Sean Marshall put it this way, "If you have spent 30 years walking into the woods, you shouldn't expect to walk out in three days." When you have spent 30 years eating a subpar diet, and dealing with an overactive mind and a non-stop lifestyle, it is unreasonable to expect that acupuncture or any other form of treatment can help after only a couple of sessions.

Acupuncture is a therapeutic process. It addresses both overt symptoms and underlying causes. Patients often need some work on underlying weaknesses in their system before any improvement in primary symptoms will manifest. The acupuncturist can spot these weaknesses, for instance insufficient fluid status, and treat to strengthen them. When you, the patient, engage in your own healing process, your health is more likely to improve. Recovery can accelerate if you concurrently make deliberate adjustments in your emotional and food diets, and/or take more time to be quiet and meditate on the state of your life and health. Another teacher of mine, Dr. Bonnie Walker, used to say, "If you keep doing the same things you've always done, you'll keep getting the same things you've always gotten."

Acupuncture therapy is a collaboration between patient and acupuncturist. Each must do their part. I have seen my patients wake up to themselves and start actively participating as they begin to notice what they feel during and between treatments. Some changes or sensations are dramatic and fast, others subtle and slow. Many patients become aware that physical symptoms are being caused by a particular stressor or component of their diet. These realizations lead them to take a more active role in the control and guidance of their own life and healing.

For health issues endured over many years, an initial six to ten treatments may be needed before any real progress can be made. Three treatments within the first two weeks helps create momentum in the body's self-healing process. After that, weekly sessions are recommended until improvement can be sustained for a full week. Finally, spreading the treatments to every two, then three weeks, and eventually progressing to a tune-up every three months, will allow the chronic sufferer to achieve and maintain a state of well-being.

The aforementioned regimens are merely my recommendations after years of observation and experience treating many patients. If you cannot follow a regular course of multiple treatments, don't let that dissuade you from trying acupuncture. I have seen its effect in a variety of scenarios.

I have seen improvement with patients who could not keep a regular schedule whether it was due to financial constraints, work-life calendar conflicts, or transportation issues. We have proceeded sometimes on a random, widely-spaced course of treatment. Since acupuncture treats the cause as well as the symptoms of illness, each treatment has long-lasting effect. Single or scattered treatments have produced tremendous results for many patients. Even one treatment could change your life.

Each patient's process with acupuncture is much like the voyage of a large ship. If that ship is already underway from New York to Hamburg and the captain receives a directive to change their destination to Barcelona, they must change course. This entails making a fair number of course corrections. These corrections are generally a series of small changes in direction at various points along the chosen route. Each small turn has lasting impact on the route taken.

Similarly each acupuncture treatment has a lasting effect on your course through life. One person's journey away from his port of origin, called illness, to a destination port, called health, might require more maneuvering on the departure end, like the complex maneuvering out of New York Harbor. Another voyage may have very few turns in the early part of the route, but require more frequent course corrections mid-journey when they encounter a storm. Yet another may require only occasional course corrections at widely spaced intervals en route to their destination port. Each treatment is a little correction that has lasting impact.

IN SUMMARY:
- The number of acupuncture treatments required for each patient or each ailment varies considerably.
- Patients often reach plateaus in their healing process due to the protective pattern of their bodies.
- Young patients often respond quickly to acupuncture.
- Monthly treatments are helpful for anyone experiencing ongoing physical or emotional stress.
- Older patients respond well to weekly or bi-monthly treatments.
- Treatment with acupuncture is not *magic*; it is a therapeutic process often involving long courses of treatment.
- For health issues endured over many years, an initial six to ten treatments may be needed before any real progress can be made.

CHAPTER 7

Do I Have To Be on a Special Diet?

You do not have to change your diet for acupuncture to work. The diagnostic process of Chinese medicine takes you just as you are in your present state. However, your acupuncturist can offer some dietary suggestions that may be of great benefit.

Patients traditionally get very little information from their doctors about diet. This is because the focus of modern medical training is on diagnosis and treatment, not the cause of disease. Diet can be both a bane and a boon to health. An improper diet can cause many physical problems, just as a healthy diet can support and enhance well-being. Unfortunately, medical doctors receive little to no training in nutrition, and since most patients will only make a change in their diet if their doctor suggests it, this can easily prolong their poor condition. Add the plethora of false and misleading marketing messages we see plastered on the packaging of grocery store products that claim to be "healthy" or "all natural," and it's hard to determine what really is beneficial to eat.

The research that determines what defines proper diet, health, and nutrition is constantly changing. The scientification of food has not always been helpful to our health. Many studies are conducted improperly, are biased, skewed or based on small samples. How many times have we heard the industry reverse its position on a food? In a natural system as complex as a human being, it is folly to use causal analysis to determine that one factor is creating one problem. Eggs are bad for us, then they're good for us, then they're bad again. Similar contradictions can be found about milk, red wine, coffee...the list goes on. The bottom line is that nutrition is complex, and the food we consume has complex effects on how we feel. It affects our physical and emotional health in ways that continue to surprise us.

We really have two diets, our **food diet** and our **emotional diet**.

Food Diet – The word "diet" in Western culture is most often associated with a short-term adjustment in our eating habits to achieve weight loss. If the foods you consume need constant monitoring and correction, you are most likely not eating a "healthy diet."

More correctly though, diet means a sustainable way of eating that creates and perpetuates health. Such a diet requires few, if any, short-term corrections. A person may adjust their intake temporarily when they are ill, for example, eating more soup if they feel chilled, or drinking more fluids if they are dehydrated. Food can be medicinal.

So what should we eat? This topic has filled an untold number of volumes, and has spawned a mega-industry. It is impossible to sort through all the varied opinions about what constitutes a healthy diet. When reduced to the simplest concept, the quality and quantity of what you eat or drink can affect your health for good or bad. Many of the products available in our grocery stores are designed for convenience and profit. They are food-like substances (processed foods), not real food (food in its natural state). Our body perceives these unhealthy edibles not as food but as foreign toxins, and responds with its immune system. Continuously challenging our immune system with a diet heavy in unnatural, processed foods will make us tired, weak, and progressively more ill. No medical treatment can overcome the relentless assault that a commercial diet has on your body. Quite simply, you may not get well if you continue to eat as you always have.

Cultivating a diet to improve your health begins by eliminating foods that can cause inflammation and adding foods to combat inflammation. I encourage you to start your own exploration by researching "inflammatory foods" and "anti-inflammatory diet." I have seen significant positive impact on my patients' health when they made a few culinary changes based on these two concepts. Once you have removed inflammatory foods from your diet, and have added back some anti-inflammatories, I encourage you to go even further. Try adding more whole foods, and see for yourself the positive effects a few simple changes can make in how good you feel. You can win back a new meaning of diet.

Food can be a healer. This is where Chinese medical dietary theory has a vast amount of knowledge and wisdom to offer. For the best, most readable book available on this topic, I suggest, *Welcoming Food: Diet as Medicine for Home Cooks and Other Healers*. This book was written by my teacher and friend, Andrew Sterman, who has immersed himself in the study of Chinese food therapy for over 20 years.

The food we choose to eat can be very personal. It often feels sacred. Certain foods give us a sense of comfort and security. Our food preferences are often based on what we were served at home, family values, or cultural practices we grew up with. We like to think that what we have always eaten is just fine and can't possibly be contributing to our health problems. It is a difficult reality to face when this simply is not true.

For many Americans, the number one factor driving our choice of food today is convenience. Eating robs us of our time to be productive. Many of us have become conditioned to just grab a bite on-the-go, or to eat our meals in front of the television or at our desks. Sharing time together as a family over a daily sit-down, home-made dinner has been relegated to holidays and special occasions. Food is more than fuel; it is also builds families and strengthens cultural bonds. When we place less importance on meal time and healthy eating practices, the vitality of the family unit and community suffers.

Emotional Diet – Our emotional diet has a direct impact on our physical health and well-being. Just like our food diet, we ingest the emotional input of our world; we chew on it, digest it, assimilate and eliminate it. Ideally, we express our feelings about life's stressors on a regular basis, and release that tension instead of storing it.

We have all experienced an emotional imposition on our physical well-being. Who hasn't had digestive upset, nausea, "butterflies," indigestion, or diarrhea as the result of being scared, nervous or angry? We inherently know our emotions affect us physically.

When this happens, it is worthwhile to examine your emotional diet. It is seductively easy to succumb to the fear and anger inherent in our incessant media feed. We barely realize that we are saturating our protective channels (Luo and Divergent) with emotions that we can't digest and don't eliminate. We slowly become alienated from our own sensibilities, in a state of denial that we are stressed, angry, scared, sad, or overwhelmed. We just keep soldiering along. Because these channels hold unexpressed emotions in the limbs and joints, we often develop pain, dysfunction, and degeneration in these areas. The protective channels traverse our entire body, externally and internally, so any one of a multitude of internal medical dysfunctions can develop from these stored emotions. This is how emotional stress contributes to physical disease. In closing, I will offer you one case study about the effect of food diet on a patient's health.

CASE STUDY

A while ago I had my first appointment with a war veteran. His wife accompanied him and they were both very interested in acupuncture and were actively engaged with the process. I explained that certain foods can cause inflammation, and that ice-cold drinks are also damaging to digestion and health, so they decided to experiment. They eliminated some of the inflammatory foods they were eating regularly, and added some anti-inflammatory foods to their diet. They reduced their consumption of iced tea and iced water. Within three weeks, he had lost six pounds, and reduced his waistline by several inches. He no longer felt bloated. She experienced significantly-reduced abdominal pain and bloating, and had so much energy that she felt good enough to mow her three-acre yard in one day.

It's amazing how only slight adjustments to your diet, and maintaining a warm digestive tract can improve your health so rapidly. When the challenge of immune-stimulating foods is removed, your system self-regulates back to its normal, healthy function.

CHAPTER 8

How Do I Find an Acupuncturist?

Acupuncture involves the insertion of needles into your body, so it is important, first and foremost, that you trust your acupuncturist. Besides licensed acupuncturists, there are many other medically-trained professionals who practice this art: doctors, osteopaths, chiropractors, physician assistants, registered nurses, nurse practitioners, dentists, and physical therapists. The degree of training and level of qualification varies by profession, though, so you'll want to investigate how thorough your acupuncturist's training really is before engaging in treatments with him or her.

Acupuncture Training Required by Profession

Licensed Acupuncturists – As of this writing, 48 states in the U.S. have acupuncture licensing boards. To practice legally in those states, an acupuncturist must have a state license. To qualify for a license, an acupuncturist must:

- Complete a 4-year master's degree or diploma-granting course of study at a school accredited by the ACAOM (Accreditation Commission for Acupuncture and Oriental Medicine). This includes 2,198 academic course hours for a total of 119 course credits. The curriculum includes advanced anatomy and physiology, pathophysiology, in-depth study of the qualitative organizational models of Chinese medicine, familiarity with clean-needle technique, and a full year of clinical practice in the school clinic under the oversight of a licensed acupuncturist.

- Pass a professional board exam administered by either the NCCAOM (National Certification Commission for Acupuncture and Oriental Medicine) or, in California, the state licensing board. This is a rigorous, comprehensive exam like those required for obtaining a medical, law, or engineering license.

- Apply for and be granted a license to practice by a state acupuncture licensing board.

Anyone who has persevered through this education and testing process certainly has the knowledge to treat you safely and effectively.

There is a substantial difference between the superficial knowledge of a subject and the deeper wisdom that comes from years of hands-on experience and insight gained over time of the things that cannot be taught. There is more to acupuncture than simply sticking needles into patients. When you embark on any new experience—especially one as intimate as seeing a new doctor or professional who will be treating your body, mind and spirit—it's important that you approach treatment with an open mind that is tuned-in to the practitioner you are considering for treatment. Recognize if you have a good or bad feeling about that person based on first impressions, and trust your "gut."

When you see any health practitioner for the first time, ask yourself the following questions: Do they really listen to you? Do they respect your intuition about what you think is wrong with you? Do they maintain eye contact? Do they pressure you into services or treatments that you don't feel you need or didn't ask for? Are they in a rush to see the next patient? These are important considerations to assess your comfort level before moving forward. How do you FEEL about that person and their practice?

Review the models of Chinese medicine in Chapter 4. This is a holistic medicine that considers your complete makeup—physical, emotional, and spiritual. Acupuncture treatment, as all medical treatments, touches us deeply, so take care in choosing your practitioner.

Due to the current opioid addiction crisis, modern medicine is losing one of their go-to tools for pain management. A large cross-section of physicians and other medical professionals are now looking to acupuncture to fill the void. Acupuncture is widely known for its effectiveness in treating pain, but it can also treat other directly- or indirectly-related symptoms as well as the addiction problem.

For consumer information and safety reasons it is important that you know the qualifications of a practitioner proposing to give you acupuncture. The following list shows the training and legal requirements for various modern medical professionals to practice acupuncture:

Medical doctors and osteopaths – Some medical doctors and osteopaths utilize acupuncture. Their requirements for practicing acupuncture vary depending on what their state medical license allows as scope-of-practice. Most states include acupuncture in a medical doctor's scope-of-practice. Others require a 300- to 350-hour course. Some require a separate license from their acupuncture licensing board, meaning that they must have the same Chinese medical education as a licensed acupuncturist. Some physicians pursue a true Chinese medical education and are highly-skilled acupuncturists. Others know just enough to "stick it where it hurts." I applaud any modern medical practitioner with the courage and dedication to study Chinese medical theory. The American Academy of Medical Acupuncture caters solely to physicians and other modern medical practitioners. Its goal is to offer the highest level of care available to patients by providing acupuncture as an alternative medical intervention, since it has a low rate of adverse side effects.

Chiropractors – Chiropractors have different requirements to practice acupuncture depending on their state's law. The criteria range from the inclusion of acupuncture in their scope-of-practice; to requiring a 100- to 300-hour course, plus exam; to obtaining a separate acupuncture license. Some states allow them to practice dry needling with or without training. (See Physical Therapy requirements below.) Like medical doctors, some chiropractors have completed an in-depth Chinese medical education and are highly skilled acupuncturists.

Registered nurses, nurse practitioners, physician assistants – This group generally cannot practice acupuncture legally without becoming a licensed acupuncturist.

U.S. military personnel – The U.S. Department of Defense has three tiers of acupuncture practice. In 2008 they began training medics and others in a simple form of ear acupuncture, which they call Battlefield Acupuncture, used for acute pain control in a combat theater. Also, some branches of the military now provide access to a 300-hour medical acupuncture training course for their physicians and physician assistants. Both of these may only be practiced within a military environment. Finally, the Department of Veterans Affairs (VA) recently began adding licensed acupuncturists to their staff, and are contracting licensed acupuncturists outside the VA system to service their veterans due to high demand.

Dentists – Dentistry is another field of medicine that is using acupuncture as alternative pain control. UCLA offers an 80-hour course for dentists covering rudimentary Chinese medical theory and application of acupuncture to the mouth and head. Some states consider acupuncture within the scope-of-practice of dentistry.

Physical therapists – Depending on a state's scope-of-practice definition, physical therapists are now able to administer "dry needling." PTs adopted the term proclaiming it to be a modern discovery, but it is actually acupuncture. Their technique addresses tight, painful areas, called "trigger points," within the muscles. Acupuncturists have been practicing similar methods for over 2,000 years. They refer to these "trigger points" as *ashi points* (stagnation of the energy channels), and use the same solid filiform needles used by physical therapists today.

Physical therapists have added acupuncture to their therapeutic toolbox, even though they are not required to undergo the same training requirements as medical doctors, chiropractors, or licensed acupuncturists. The minimum requirement for physical therapists to achieve "dry needling" certification is completion of a continuing-education course between 46-54 hours. This is the first exposure in their professional training to the use of either solid or hypodermic needles, both considered invasive procedures. While physical therapy's general scope-of-practice includes the application of topical and aerosol treatments, it does not typically include drug prescription or injection of any kind. Physical therapists are not even certified to perform finger sticks for basic capillary blood testing.

Such a minimal educational requirement to perform an invasive medical procedure presents a significant risk to public safety. By contrast, a licensed acupuncturist's training includes a concentrated focus, reinforced by a full year of supervised clinical practice on which points and anatomical locations present a risk of internal injury should a needle be inserted too deeply. For example, deep-needle insertion to the thorax increases the risk of causing collapsed lung (pneumothorax). A significant number of these injuries have been documented in instances where the physical therapist did not have sufficient training to understand the implications of deep needle insertion in this area.

In 2016, the American Medical Association (AMA) adopted a policy that said physical therapists and other non-physicians practicing dry needling should, at a minimum, have standards similar to the training, certification and continuing education standards that exist for licensed acupuncturists.

In a June 15, 2016 AMA press release entitled, "AMA Adopts New Policies on Final Day of Annual Meeting," AMA Board Member Russell W. H. Kridel, M.D. stated that, "Lax regulation and nonexistent standards surround this invasive practice. For patients' safety, practitioners should meet standards required for licensed acupuncturists and physicians."

In summary, carefully consider the training and qualifications of any practitioner you allow to give you acupuncture. Don't be afraid to ask for proof of training if you do not see a certificate or license displayed on the wall.

CONCLUSION

To conclude, I thought it would be helpful to describe the typical flow of an acupuncture session for those who have never tried it. A visit to your acupuncturist is much like a visit to your medical doctor. The one exception is, during your appointment, you will receive treatment that actively helps you. There is no waiting for test results or having to pick up a prescription before beginning therapy. You will leave your acupuncturist's office feeling some level of change after each session.

There are two general practice types. The first is more like the modern medical model where each patient is seen individually in a private treatment room. The second, called Community Acupuncture, has multiple patients being treated simultaneously in a larger setting at reduced cost to the patient. Most folks have a clear preference for one setting over the other. Acupuncture offices are often decorated in a way that is soothing and nurturing to the soul. A beautiful, relaxed environment is much more conducive to healing than a bland, clinical, impersonal examining room.

On your initial visit to my office, there is some paperwork to complete first. It will request contact information, chief health complaint, a list of current medications, short medical history, HIPAA privacy notice, an informed consent, and an arbitration agreement.

Each appointment is typically an hour long. I prefer scheduling your next appointment and procuring payment up-front so that you can leave at the end of your treatment feeling relaxed with a sense of well-being, uninterrupted by a business transaction.

It is often a good idea to use the bathroom before a treatment session. You'll want to feel comfortable, with no distractions during needling. Treatment begins with me asking about your current state-of-health, any changes from the last treatment, and assessment of your appearance, the sound of your voice, and your energetic pulses. This is the diagnostic process—a careful synthesis of different factors that tells me which channels and acupuncture points to treat during this visit. Treatment points may be different with each visit, or they may be the same.

How much you need to disrobe will be based on access needed to the channels and points to be treated. Undressing down to underwear is sometimes necessary, but often removal of just shoes and socks and either shirt or pants is sufficient. To preserve modesty, I have shorts and loose coverings available. Everything described to this point takes about 15 to 20 minutes.

The treatment table is very similar to a massage table to create a comfortable, safe and relaxed feeling. Depending on the channels and points being treated, you will lie face-up, face-down, or on your side. Some treatments require a change of position part way through. For example, you may begin the session face-down for moxa (or cupping) on your back, then turn and lie on your back so needles may be inserted on your front. (See Fig. 17.)

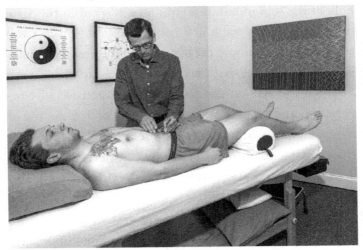

Fig. 17 Patient Treatment

Needle insertion generally takes five minutes or less. With each needle, I have you breathe in, and on the exhale, I slip the needle into the acupuncture point. This helps create a level of comfort and predictability so you aren't surprised by the insertion of the next needle.

Once the needling is complete, you are covered with a space blanket for warmth. This is a lightweight, foil blanket that is used to retain heat in emergency situations. It is so light that it does not interfere with the needles. Covering you with the blanket also gives you a sense of security and privacy. This is to encourage the healing process. At this point, I will leave the room while the needles do their job. You will have a call button in case you need assistance or require anything, like water or emotional support. The bulk of the session, 20 to 30 minutes, is spent in this state of warmth and relaxation. When the session is over, I will come back in to remove the blanket and the needles. Finally, you are free to get dressed and leave at a leisurely pace.

That's it! As you can see, your hour consists of conversation and treatment. Treatments involving the use of moxa, cupping, or Gua Sha require more hands-on time than treatments using only needles. Either way, you will leave a changed person—less anxious, with less pain, and deeply relaxed.

I sincerely appreciate your interest in acupuncture and thank you for taking the time to explore it in greater depth with me. I too have learned even more about my practice by revisiting the many concepts of Chinese medicine through the writing process. I still find the ancient Eastern theories fascinating and complex. They continue to teach me a great deal about myself. I trust that with some time and reflection, they will do the same for you.

Glossary and Pronunciation Guide

Acupressure – finger pressure applied in lieu of needles to activate acupuncture points.

Anatomy and Physiology – the branch of biology concerned with the study of the structure of organisms and their parts.

Chi \ chē \ – energy

Chinese Medicine – medical system of healthcare based on the concepts of Chi or energy, employing Yin/Yang, Five Phases, Phase Associations, and Energy Channels as its organizational models. Its therapeutic tools include acupuncture, cupping, gua sha, moxa, massage and herbal prescriptions.

Cupping – a technique used in conjunction with acupuncture involving placement of suction cups to pull positive pressure on tissue to unblock stagnation in the energy channels.

Daoism \ daủ-i-zəm, taủ- \ – Chinese philosophical system dating from around 400 BCE.

Deqi \ dā-kē \ – The sensation felt after an acupuncture needle is inserted. It usually does not persist and is the excitation of the energy or Chi in the energy channels.

Disease-Management Approach – healthcare based on diagnosis and treatment of material disease. This is the model of modern medicine.

Electrical Stimulation – use of a microcurrent device in lieu of needles to activate acupuncture points. Also the use of microcurrent applied via electrical leads attached to needles.

Energetic System – the unseen, unmeasurable circulatory system of energy in the human body composed of five classes of energy channels.

Energy Channels (also called Acupuncture Channels or Meridians) – conduits of the unseen electromagnetic energy, or Chi, that circulates in the human body and underlies all form and function.

Five Phases (also know as Five Elements) – one of the organizational models of Chinese medical theory that qualitatively describes the laws of nature and the functional relationships between the organ systems of the human being.

**Gua Sha \ gwä-shä ** – a technique used in conjunction with acupuncture involving scraping of the skin (Gua) causing a deep redness (Sha) to rises to the surface. This unblocks stagnation in the energy channels restoring circulation and reducing pain.

Luo \ lō \ – connecting; also the name of one class of acupuncture channel.

Macrocosm – the largest view of a subject

Microcosm – a small subset of the whole

Modern Medicine – medical system of healthcare based on germ theory and employing biology and biochemistry as its organizational models. Its therapeutic tools include pharmacology, surgery, and physical therapy.

Moxa \ mäk-sə \ – A therapeutic tool used in some acupuncture treatments utilizing the plant mugwort rolled into cigar form or placed loosely on top of a needle, which is burned to induce warmth into the energy channels.

Pathophysiology – the branch of biology that examines the malfunction of physiological processes that lead to disease or injury.

Pulse and Tongue Diagnosis – two assessment tools used in the diagnostic process in Chinese medicine.

Qualitative – assessment of a thing or being based on its essential nature.

Quantitative – assessment of a thing or being based on material measurement.

Shen \ shin \ – the spirit of a person

BURTON MOOMAW

Tai Chi \ tī-chē, tī-jē \ – an internal martial art practiced for cultivation of health and for defensive purposes.

Wei Chi \ wā-chē \ – the body's defensive energy, most closely equating to the concept of the immune system.

Yang \ yaNG, yäNG, yaŋ \ – the light half of the Taijitu or Yin/Yang symbol. It represents light, energy, and function, among other descriptors.

Yang Energy – active or functional energy

Yin \ yin, yiŋ \ – the dark half of the Taijitu or Yin/Yang symbol. It represents darkness, material, and form, among other descriptors.

Yin Energy – material or structural energy

Ying Chi \yin-chē, yiŋ-chē \ – the body's fuel energy, most closely equating to the concept of the oxygen and food nutrients that circulate in our blood.

Yuan Chi \ yü-ən chē, yü-än chē \ – the body's ancestral energy, most closely equating to the concept of DNA.

103

Index

F

G

H

I

K

L

M

N

O

P

Q

R

Acknowledgments

I would like to acknowledge and thank the following for their contributions to this book:

All of my patients for the privilege of sharing your lives.

Julia Rechenbach-Moomaw, my wife, for always allowing and encouraging me to stay out of the box.

Franklin and Mary Kathryn Moomaw for their love and support.

Betty Kirkpatrick for her prodding questions and unending encouragement.

My teachers: Dr. Sean Marshall, Dr. Bonnie Walker, Dr. Tran Viet Tzung, Jeffery Yuen, Ann Cecil-Sterman, and Andrew Sterman, for your many contributions to my life.

Curt O'Briant and Ged Moody for their title suggestions.

Susan Yost, editor extraordinaire and layout wizard, for her skill with language and helping me clarify my ideas.

Courtney Tiberio of FullSteam Labs, for cover and image creation, and her publishing expertise.

Todd Bush for his refined photography skills.

Justin Simmons for being a photo model.

Marie Bongiovanni and Valerie Doebley for proofreading the final draft.

Kathryn Kirkpatrick for proofreading and index development.

Jung Tao School of Classical Chinese Medicine, my alma mater, for permission to use their copyrighted images.

Author Bio

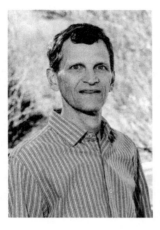

BURTON MOOMAW lives and practices in Boone, NC. He was drawn to study acupuncture after witnessing it support his wife's second pregnancy when she was struggling with hypothyroidism and infertility. He received a diploma of acupuncture from Jung Tao School of Classical Chinese Medicine in Sugar Grove, NC and now serves on the school's board of directors. His continuing education led him to study extensively with Jeffrey Yuen and Ann Cecil-Sterman to deepen his knowledge of the channels of acupuncture.

Burton was a founding owner of the rock climbing gear manufacturer Misty Mountain Threadworks and the first professionally certified rock climbing guide in the southeastern USA. He lives with his German-born wife of 30 years, Julia Rechenbach-Moomaw, and is the proud father of Lucas and Noah Moomaw.

Made in the USA
Columbia, SC
29 April 2020